God Wants You Well

by
Andrew Wommack

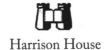

Harrison House

24 23 22   20 19 18

God Wants You Well
ISBN 13: 978-1-60683-004-8
ISBN 10: 1-60683-004-X
Copyright © 2010 by Andrew Wommack Ministries, Inc.
850 Elkton Dr.
Colorado Springs, CO 80907

Published by Harrison House Publishers
www.harrisonhouse.com

Contents

Introduction

Chapter 1 Miracles Confirm God's Word.................................1

Chapter 2 Part of His Atonement..9

Chapter 3 Sozo!...15

Chapter 4 The Full Package 21

Chapter 5 Sickness and Sin..31

Chapter 6 A Cop Out..39

Chapter 7 Paul's Thorn in the Flesh.....................................49

Chapter 8 Eye Problems? 61

Chapter 9 Redeemed from the Curse....................................69

Chapter 10 Jesus Healed Them All.......................................79

Chapter 11 Why Isn't Everyone Healed? 85

Chapter 12 "Because of Your Unbelief"................................95

Chapter 13 Faith Negated...105

Chapter 14 A Pure, Strong Faith 115

Chapter 15 Governed by Law 127

Chapter 16 The Spiritual World 137

Chapter 17 Words Are Powerful...147

Chapter 18 Act on Your Faith 159

My Prayer for Your Healing 169

Is It Always God's Will to Heal?..171

Scriptures..173

Recommended Teachings...207

Endnotes 209

Introduction

Although I don't know everything there is to know about healing, I have grown a lot in this area, and consider it to be a real strength in my life. In fact, it's now been almost forty years since I've had sickness win in my body. That doesn't mean I've never had a problem. Along the way, I've had things attack me. One time, while I was making radio programs, all of the symptoms of the flu hit me. My sinuses stopped up, my nose ran, and I began to have aches, chills, and fever—all within a very short period of time. It took me about an hour praying over it, but then it was gone.

Probably one of the worst sicknesses that's come against me these past forty years[1] was the time I returned home from England and went right to work on my pond. Although I'd gone thirty-four hours without sleep, something had happened with the drain in the pond I was building on my property, so I had to attend to it immediately. Standing chest deep in cold water and working for about six hours while I was so weak, tired, and depleted was not smart on my part. Soon my nose began to run and my ears plugged up, yet I was able to overcome that runny nose in just about a day's time. Although it took me a couple of days to get my ears unplugged, an outside observer probably wouldn't have been able to tell that anything had occurred.

That's the worst illness that I can remember dealing with in almost forty years. At the very beginning of this period of time,

I was actually diagnosed with an incurable disease. However, within three days that same doctor pronounced me whole because I had received prayer and healing. So I've seen God heal me of a number of things.

Healing is a strength in my life. These truths I share in this book are working for me, and have been for decades. Even though I don't understand everything there is to understand about healing, I know more than I'll be able to talk about in this message. Please refer to the "Recommended Teachings" section for additional resources that will complement and expand on the truths contained here. My purpose in this book isn't to teach healing in an exhaustive manner, but to lay a firm foundation.

How About You?

You need to consider the truths of God's Word contained in this book. Although I've personally walked in divine health for a long time, it's not because nothing has ever happened to me. I've been hurt, had accidents, and been attacked by sickness. I've had problems, but I've overcome them—and I've seen good health manifest in my own physical body for decades.

I've also ministered healing to multitudes of others. I've seen the blind receive sight. This includes both partially blind eyes that improved and totally blind eyes—that couldn't even perceive light—opened. I've seen both totally and partially deaf people hear. I remember praying for people whose eardrums had deteriorated, or had even been surgically removed. God restored their hearing. I've seen individuals who couldn't even talk because their larynx was gone receive a miracle and start speaking in tongues. I've seen thousands of people healed of arthritis and all kinds of pain. One man had a metal rod in his back that made him stand up straight. It was physically impossible for him to bend over, yet he received healing and bent over just fine. I've seen deformities healed, diseases cured, and people come out of wheelchairs.

I've personally seen three people raised from the dead, including my own son. He'd been dead for almost five hours, and had already turned black. His toe was tagged and he was lying on a slab in the hospital morgue, but the Lord raised him up—glory to His name!

I don't share any of this to promote myself. I'm still learning about healing. There have been—and still are—times when I pray for people and they aren't healed. But I'm getting better results today than ever before. I haven't arrived, but I've left, and I've learned some important truths along the way.

How about you? Are you consistently walking in divine health? Are the people you pray for regularly healed? If not, then you ought to seriously consider the truths I'm sharing.

God's Word Works

Please don't mistake my confidence for arrogance, but this is an area of my life where I've seen results. I've personally ministered to probably hundreds of thousands of people. I've trained others and seen these truths work for them. A lot of ministers have told me how receiving a revelation of these same truths has enabled them to see many people they have prayed for healed. Some of these ministers have seen nearly every single individual they prayed for healed, including multiple people raised from the dead. God's Word works!

I may not have it all figured out, but I know I'm going in the right direction. I've seen the power of God work again and again. If you're prejudiced against healing and refuse to consider what the Word says, I probably won't be able to help you. But if you genuinely desire to know about the divine healing that is available through the Lord Jesus Christ and faith in what He's done, this book could literally change your life. At the very least, these truths can bring you to a level of success and victory in this area of healing equal to what God has given me. Again, I don't claim to have arrived, but healing is manifesting itself in my life—not only just for me, but also for the people to whom I've been ministering.

As you humble yourself to receive God's Word, I believe these truths will really help you too.

Chapter 1

Miracles Confirm God's Word

Many people criticize me for emphasizing healing. They say, "This isn't important. You don't have to be healed to go to heaven. You shouldn't spend any of your time on radio, television, or in print emphasizing healing. It's a secondary issue. You're making it greater than it is."

One of the radio stations my program is broadcast on forwarded me a letter awhile back from a man who threatened to take legal action against me. Basically, he said, "It's a big sin for you to take people's money, which is hard to come by, and preach something like healing!" This fellow was one of many people who contend that it's a waste of time to talk about healing. I strongly disagree.

Healing is part of Christ's atonement. If Jesus died to provide healing for us, then it's not just incidental. If the Lord suffered and took stripes on His back for our physical healing, then it's not insignificant. If Jesus thought enough of healing to purchase it for us, then we ought to think enough of it to receive.

God the Father caused His Son to bear all of our sins and all of our sicknesses on the cross. Jesus took our diseases just as much as He took our sins. Therefore, it honors Him to promote healing. In fact, Jesus spent more time talking about healing than He did several other truths that many people consider to be essential issues today—heaven and hell in particular. Actually, the Lord used healing like a bell to get people's attention and to prove that He did have power on earth to forgive sins. Many scriptural examples illustrate this.

Healing and Forgiveness

In Mark 2, some friends of a man who suffered from the palsy couldn't get him into the house Jesus was ministering at because of the great crowd. Undeterred, they took him up to the top of the house, removed some tiles from the ceiling, and literally lowered this man in his stretcher right down in front of Jesus.

> *When Jesus saw their faith, he said unto the sick of the palsy, Son, thy sins be forgiven thee.*
>
> *Mark 2:5*

Notice that He said, "Son, your sins be forgiven you."

> *But there were certain of the scribes sitting there, and reasoning in their hearts, Why doth this man thus speak blasphemies? who can forgive sins but God only? And immediately when Jesus perceived in his spirit that they so reasoned within themselves, he said unto them, Why reason ye these things in your hearts? Whether is it easier to say to the sick of the palsy, Thy sins be forgiven thee; or to say, Arise, and take up thy bed, and walk?*
>
> *Mark 2:6–9*

If Jesus had been only a mere man, it would have been impossible for Him to say either, "Rise up and walk," or "Your sins are forgiven you." Only God can forgive sins, and man in his physical ability does not have the power to produce healing. However, Jesus being both fully God and fully Man, could actually say and provide both these things—healing and forgiveness.

It's easier to say, "Your sins be forgiven you," because you can't see a sin, and you can't see if a sin is forgiven and dealt with or not. If someone challenged you saying, "You can't do that," you could just answer, "Prove it!"

Verification

Jesus was saying that it's easier to say, "Your sins are forgiven" than "Rise up and walk" because they would immediately be able to tell if Jesus had the power to make this declaration by whether this man rose up and walked. Instantly there would be physical evidence that it did or didn't work.

The reasoning followed that if you can do the greater work, then certainly you can do the lesser. If you can jump fifteen feet, then certainly you can jump two feet.

The people were just standing there in silence not knowing how to respond. Then Jesus continued saying:

But that ye may know that the Son of man hath power on earth to forgive sins, (he saith to the sick of the palsy,) I say unto thee, Arise, and take up thy bed, and go thy way into thine house. And immediately he arose, took up the bed, and went forth before them all; insomuch that they were all amazed, and glorified God, saying, We never saw it on this fashion.

Mark 2:10–12

Jesus made it very clear that the reason He healed this man was so that people would know that He also had power on earth to forgive sins. The Lord used healing as a verification that He had power to deal with unseen things. If He could deal with physical bodies, and meet the physical and emotional needs of people, then He could also deal with their spiritual needs. Jesus used healing like a bell to draw people to Himself and get their attention, and then He would tell them the truth.

Words Only?

Jesus also said that the miracles He did authenticated who He was and confirmed what He said.

I have greater witness than that of John: for the works which the Father hath given me to finish, the same works that I do, bear witness of me, that the Father hath sent me.

John 5:36

Although Jesus pointed to the testimony that John the Baptist bore of Him, He wasn't counting on it. Christ was dependent on the confirmation His Father gave of who He was by the miracles He performed. If Jesus needed the witness of the miracles He performed to validate His authority, then how can we possibly do less? It is the height of arrogance to think that we can use words only to persuade people when Jesus had to have signs and miracles to confirm His Word.

The Way It Should Be

Some folks say, "We don't need miracles today. We have the Word of God." Yet, that's not what the Bible teaches. Mark 16 reveals to us some of the very last instructions Jesus gave His disciples before He ascended back to heaven. Notice what He promised after commanding us to go into all the world and preach the Gospel:

> *These signs shall follow them that believe; In my name shall they cast out devils; they shall speak with new tongues; They shall take up serpents; and if they drink any deadly thing, it shall not hurt them; they shall lay hands on the sick, and they shall recover. So then after the Lord had spoken unto them, he was received up into heaven, and sat on the right hand of God. And they went forth, and preached every where, the Lord working with them, and confirming the word with signs following.*
>
> *Mark 16:17–20*

In other words, God used miracles to confirm that it was really Him speaking through these people. This scripture also reveals that the Lord confirms the true preaching and teaching of His Word with signs following.

Based on this, we can truthfully say today that if ministers do not have the miraculous power of God flowing through them, then we should be skeptical about whether or not God is truly speaking through them. Now, don't misunderstand me. I'm not saying that a person who doesn't have healings manifest in his or her ministry is not of God. Neither am I saying to just automatically trust all the words of anyone who performs a miracle. You must always check what people say against God's Word. However, in God's system, when His Word is truly preached there will be signs and wonders following.

We live in a day and age where the message of salvation has been corrupted and divided into parts. Certain aspects are neglected and misunderstood by most of the body of Christ. Many people are preaching only the forgiveness of sins. God confirms all of His Word that we preach, but if all we preach on is spiritual, eternal values, and the forgiveness of sins, then all we'll see happen is people being born again. But if we preach and teach the whole counsel of God, He will confirm it with signs, wonders, and miracles. This is the way God has established it in the scriptures, and this is the way it should be.

We Do Too!

Not every true man or woman of God sees miracles nowadays because they aren't preaching the whole counsel of God. Some people I respect very much have been faithful with the revelation that they have. They've seen people born again and lives transformed. I definitely wouldn't say that they aren't true ministers. Yet, it's obvious that they aren't preaching the whole counsel of God. God's will is for His whole counsel to be preached, and He will confirm it with signs and wonders following.

Hebrews 2:3–4 says:

How shall we escape, if we neglect so great salvation; which at the first began to be spoken by the Lord, and was confirmed unto us by them that heard him; God also bearing them witness, both with signs and wonders, and with divers miracles, and gifts of the Holy Ghost, according to his own will?

This says that God confirmed the Word that Jesus preached with miracles. When He had ascended to heaven and the disciples took over the ministry on this earth, God also confirmed the Word that they spoke with signs, wonders, and gifts of the Holy Spirit according to His will.

No one today can claim they are operating better than Jesus did. In fact, most Christians aren't even regularly seeing the fullness of the manifestation of God's power the way that the early apostles did. Who do we think that we are to believe that somehow or another we have a superior anointing or ability to minister effectively in God's eyes without needing miracles today? That's the height of arrogance. If both Jesus and the early believers needed miracles, signs, and wonders to confirm the message from God that they preached, then we do too.

Chapter 2

Part of His Atonement

If the body of Christ was fully presenting the Gospel—the whole counsel of God—we'd be making a much greater impact on the world today. God not only wants to forgive us of our sins, He also loves us dearly and desires to heal our bodies, bless us financially, and deliver us from discouragement and depression. Think about that!

One of the main reasons why the modern-day Church has been rendered so ineffective and irrelevant in many people's eyes is they've only preached that God is for the hereafter. They've made relationship with the Lord a heaven and hell issue, and haven't preached that He loves us right now. They haven't taught that God wants to give us a dynamic and absolutely victorious life at this present time. They haven't ministered healing, prosperity, or deliverance.

Some statistics I've seen have said that as much as 85 percent of the population in the United States believes that there is a God, yet only 10 to 15 percent actually attend church on a regular basis. Out of all these people who say they believe in God, would there be enough evidence to convict them if they were accused of being a Christian? There is a huge gap between the people who say that God exists and those who enjoy a vibrant relationship with Him.

Why is that? Why do so many people who know God exists not go on to obtain this intimate relationship with Him and make Him the center of their lives? Although there are probably several factors, one of the most obvious is that the Church has presented relationship with God as a heaven and hell issue. They've preached, "Just get your sins forgiven so you won't go to hell."

Truly Relevant

Even though that's true—there is a heaven to gain and a hell to lose, and you must have your sins forgiven to escape hell—most people are living in such a hell in this life that they aren't concerned with a hell in the afterlife. They're in strife, enduring divorce, suffering from sickness, and terrified of what's happening out in the world. They haven't heard or seen that the Lord deals with these issues in this life. They just think that God is for the hereafter, and they're shortsighted. They should be thinking about eternity, but they aren't because they're so occupied with trying to struggle through all of the terrible things they're facing right now. They know God exists, but they put Him off until just before they die because they don't see His relevance to their present everyday life.

What if the Church were to represent the Lord more accurately by saying, "God will heal you and keep you healthy. He'll deliver you from the depression, despair, and strife that you find yourself in. God will prosper you in a way that you could never accomplish just through your own effort." If we presented the truth that God is not only for the forgiveness of sins, but for all these other areas too, then people would see that He is truly relevant to our daily life.

If a sick person came to one of many modern-day "churches" (I use that term loosely), they'd ask, "Why are you coming to us? Go to the doctor." If a poor person came, they'd say, "Well, have you checked with the government agencies and tried welfare yet?" If someone came who was discouraged, depressed, and under some kind of demonic oppression, they'd refer them to a psychiatrist or other professional who would prescribe them some kind of a drug. But that's not the attitude God wants us to have. The Church should be meeting the needs of people! Our lack of doing so is one reason that many folks see the Church as irrelevant to their present life. They don't doubt God's existence. They just don't see why they need Him until they get ready to die. That's wrong!

Our example—Jesus—emphasized healing. I am simply following Him. Everywhere Jesus went, He healed people. God the Father used these miracles to show people that Jesus had power on earth to forgive sins. This confirmed Christ's message and proved the validity of His words. Since that's the way God did it with Jesus, I'm following a good precedent.

A terrible signal is sent both to unbelievers and Christians alike when misled preachers say things like, "God doesn't care about the healing of your body," or "He's putting sickness on you to teach you a lesson." That's absolutely untrue!

Not Just An "Add-on"

My dad died just about a month after I turned twelve. He was in a coma for a period of time before that. So I went through this grueling experience of my father being on the verge of death for months as an eleven year old. The church that I grew up in said that the Lord put that sickness on him, and it was God's will that he died. I didn't rebel against God because of that, but deep down in my heart something about it just didn't sit right.

However, I can give you examples of many other people who went through similar experiences and did rebel. One fellow is very famous. As a young boy he knew that God existed, and even sought Him. But his sister died and the religious people told him that God did it. He turned completely away from the Lord and today is a very outspoken atheist. He cites this example in his life and says, "You can't tell me that if there is a God He would put sickness on people!" This misrepresentation of God turns a lot of folks away from the Lord and embitters them against Him.

It's only the grace of God that kept me from rebelling when I was told, "God is the one who killed your dad." Many others haven't responded as well.

Countless people know God exists, but for whatever reason, they just don't want anything to do with Him, or they don't see His relevance to their everyday life. That's why healing needs to be emphasized. We need to speak the truth of the whole counsel of God. Although healing shouldn't be elevated above forgiveness of sins, neither should it be diminished below it.

Jesus provided healing for us at the same time as He provided forgiveness for our sins.

Healing isn't just an "add-on" or an "added benefit" that only happens sometimes. It's an essential part of what Christ came to do. Jesus died for the physical healing of our bodies just the same as He died for our forgiveness of sins. The Lord purchased healing for us just as He purchased forgiveness. It's all part of His atonement.

A Done Deal

This truth is not yet widely understood and believed across the body of Christ today, which explains why so few people are walking in it. Most Christians think that God could certainly heal if He wanted to, but they don't see that He has already redeemed us from sickness and disease. They view healing as something the Lord can do, but they don't know for sure that it is His will.

If you recognize that healing is part of the atonement (which took place two thousand years ago), then you'll comprehend that the Lord has already healed us. He's already purchased that blessing. That power has already been generated. Healing is a done deal, and is available to us now exactly the same as forgiveness of sins.

Chapter 3

Sozo!

[Jesus] gave himself for our sins, that he might deliver us from this present evil world, according to the will of God and our Father.

Galatians 1:4

Jesus gave Himself for our sins that He might deliver us from this present evil world—not just the evil world to come.

Many people think that what Jesus produced through His death, burial, and resurrection only affects the spiritual, eternal realm. Because of this, they come up with song lyrics referring to when all of us get to heaven, what a day it will be. Of course it will be glorious in heaven, but Jesus also came to deliver us from this present evil world. We're not just saved from hell, our sins, and future punishment—Jesus also came to deliver, protect, and provide for us in this physical world right now.

An All-Encompassing Word

The Greek word *sozo* was used over a hundred times in the New Testament. It's an all-encompassing word for salvation, often rendered "save" or "saved."[1] However, a closer look at how this important word was translated makes it very clear that our salvation includes much more than just forgiveness of sins.

Sozo was translated "save" thirty-eight times in reference to the forgiveness of sins. Some examples include:

> *She shall bring forth a son, and thou shalt call his name JESUS: for he shall save [sozo] his people from their sins.*
>
> *Matthew 1:21*

> *For after that in the wisdom of God the world by wisdom knew not God, it pleased God by the foolishness of preaching to save [sozo] them that believe.*
>
> *1 Corinthians 1:21*

> *Wherefore he is able also to save [sozo] them to the uttermost that come unto God by him, seeing he ever liveth to make intercession for them.*
>
> *Hebrews 7:25*

Forgiven, Healed, and Delivered

Sozo was translated another fifty-three times as "saved" (past tense) in reference to forgiveness of sins. However, there were also times where this exact same Greek word was translated as "healed."

> *[Jairus] besought [Jesus] greatly, saying, My little daughter lieth at the point of death: I pray thee, come and lay thy hands on her, that she may be healed [sozo]; and she shall live.*
>
> *Mark 5:23*

This word "healed" is referring to physical healing. As the story unfolds, Jairus' daughter actually died, and Jesus raised her from the dead. (Mark 5:35–43.) So in this instance *sozo*—"healed"—refers to physical healing, even physical resurrection from the dead.

This same word that's used for both forgiveness of sins and physical healing also applies to deliverance from demons.

> *They also which saw it told them by what means he that was possessed of the devils was healed [sozo].*
>
> *Luke 8:36*

Commonly called the Gadarene demoniac, nobody could hold this man. In fact, he often broke the very chains which bound him. Sometimes deliverance from demons is necessary for someone to receive healing. That is included in this word *sozo*.

> *The same heard Paul speak: who stedfastly beholding him, and perceiving that he had faith to be healed [sozo].*
>
> *Acts 14:9*

Paul beheld this crippled man and perceived that he had faith to be healed [sozo], and he was (vv. 8–10).

Christ's Saving Power

James 5:15 is a classic example of Christ's saving power manifesting in our lives both as healing and forgiveness of sins.

> *The prayer of faith shall save [sozo] the sick, and the Lord shall raise him up; and if he have committed sins, they shall be forgiven him.*

In another instance, Jesus knew the thoughts of the scribes and Pharisees, so He asked:

> *Is it lawful on the sabbath days to do good, or to do evil? to save [sozo] life, or to destroy it?*
>
> *Luke 6:9*

When they didn't answer, He turned and healed the man with the withered right hand (vv. 8–11). Jesus wasn't just talking about forgiveness of sins. He meant the healing of the body.

Made Whole

This same word—*sozo*—was also translated "made whole" in reference to healing. Consider the example of the woman with an issue of blood:

> *But Jesus turned him about, and when he saw her, he said, Daughter, be of good comfort; thy faith hath made thee whole [sozo]. And the woman was made whole [sozo] from that hour.*
>
> *Matthew 9:22*

In faith, she touched the hem of His garment and received healing. She was *sozo*—made whole. This is the same Greek word that is synonymous with forgiveness of sin. Here again, it's applied to being healed physically.

This same instance, recorded in the book of Mark, reveals that right before she reached out to Jesus, she said:

> *If I may touch but his clothes, I shall be whole [sozo].*
>
> *Mark 5:28*

Sozo!

Sozo was translated "make whole" or "be whole" eleven times in scripture. It's obvious from God's Word that salvation isn't limited only to the forgiveness of sins.

> *And whithersoever he entered, into villages, or cities, or country, they laid the sick in the streets, and besought him that they might touch if it were but the border of his garment: and as many as touched him were made whole [sozo].*
>
> *Mark 6:56*

When Jesus heard the news that Jairus' daughter had died, He answered him, saying:

> *Fear not: believe only, and she shall be made whole [sozo].*
>
> *Luke 8:50*

The Lord was referring to the healing of her physical body.

Abundantly Supplied

Salvation doesn't only mean forgiveness of sins, but includes healing of the body, deliverance, and financial prosperity, too. Many in the modern church have interpreted salvation only to be forgiveness of sins, but that's a misrepresentation of what the Lord did. Forgiveness of our sins is certainly the centerpiece, and I'm not minimizing it at all. However, at the same time Christ died to purchase our redemption from sin, He also freed us from sickness, disease, depression, and poverty.

Second Corinthians 8:9 is very clear concerning the atonement and our redemption from poverty:

*For ye know the grace of our Lord Jesus Christ, that, though
he was rich, yet for your sakes he became poor, that ye through
his poverty might be rich.*

Jesus became poor so that we through His poverty might be
made rich—abundantly supplied. Through Christ's death, burial,
and resurrection, God has provided everything we need in this life
and in the life to come—forgiveness of sins, healing, deliverance,
and prosperity. Isn't God good!

Chapter 4

The Full Package

Jesus didn't just die for our sins, and then healing was something He could do if He wanted to. No! Christ paid for the healing of our body as completely as He paid for the forgiveness of our sins. He purchased it all at once in His atonement. This may be different than what much of the modern-day church presents, but scriptures bear it out.

Consider Psalm 103:1–3, which says:

Bless the LORD, O my soul: and all that is within me, bless his holy name. Bless the LORD, O my soul, and forget not all his benefits: Who forgiveth all thine iniquities; who healeth all thy diseases.

Verse 2 specifically tells us not to forget all of His benefits. The Lord forgives all of our iniquities and heals all of our diseases (v. 3). In the New Testament, 1 Peter 2:24 agrees, saying:

Who his own self bare our sins in his own body on the tree, that we, being dead to sins, should live unto righteousness: by whose stripes ye were healed.

Both Psalm 103:3 and 1 Peter 2:24 mention the salvation benefits of forgiveness of sins and physical healing together in the same verse. Scripture does not separate what Jesus did in the atonement. Only men do that. As far as God is concerned, salvation is a package deal.

Fringe Benefits?

It's people who have said, "Let's not talk about healing, deliverance, or prosperity. Let's just focus on forgiveness of sins. That's the part that everyone can agree on. That's the main part of the atonement. All these others are just fringe benefits." Fringe benefits? I believe that's offensive to God!

Suppose I had done all the things for you that Jesus did for us—died for your sins to be forgiven, borne stripes on my body to produce healing for you, been separated from God my Father so that you would never have to be separated, became poor so that through my poverty you might be made rich. Then you came up to me and said, "Thank you for what you did, but I'm only going to take one-fourth of it. Forgiveness of sins is the most important, and that's what I really want to focus on. So I'm not going to take advantage of the healing for my body, the deliverance from demonic oppression, or the financial blessing. I just don't want those things. You did more than enough for me, so I'm going to humble myself and only take one-fourth of what you provided." It sure wouldn't bless me for you to break it up in pieces.

That wouldn't please me. It would make me feel like, "What was the point in me suffering for these other things if you aren't going to take advantage of them?"

God so loved the world that He gave His only begotten

Son (John 3:16). It wasn't only so that people wouldn't go to hell. Jesus saved us from sin, sickness, disease, and poverty. He gave Himself as the perfect atoning sacrifice that He might deliver us from this present evil world. (Galatians 1:4.)

It wouldn't please me for you to only take advantage of a small portion of everything I had suffered, bled, died, and resurrected to provide for you. If I could be like God, I'm sure that I'd still love you, but I wouldn't be pleased. I'm not saying that God is angry with people, but I'm sure He finds it disappointing that He provided all of this for us and so many of us simply aren't taking advantage of it.

Basically, Christianity has preached, "Forgiveness of sins is all that Jesus atoned for. Of course, since God is God, He could heal if He wants to, but that's like icing on the cake. That's extra. It isn't part of the basic package." No, God's Word clearly reveals that healing is an integral part of the salvation package. Healing is in the atonement just as much as forgiveness of sins!

Actively Fight Against

Once you get this revelation firmly established in your heart, it'll cause you to reject this false teaching that says, "God is the One who causes people to die. He puts sickness on you to humble you for some redemptive purpose and to perfect you through all this suffering." No! Jesus died for the forgiveness of your sins and for the healing of your body. They're all part of one complete and finished atonement. This means that Jesus would no more put sickness on you than He would lead you to sin. When you get this attitude, you'll say, "I won't submit to sickness any more than I would go out and yield to sin." Once you get that mindset, you'll start seeing healing manifest in your body.

One reason people don't see a greater degree of healing is that they aren't committed to it. They embrace infirmity thinking, *Well, this is just natural.* Even worse, many times they're told, "It's God making you sick." James 4:7 says:

Submit yourselves therefore to God. Resist the devil, and he will flee from you.

The word resist means to "actively fight against."[1] How can you actively fight against the devil—and the sickness, infirmity, and disease that come from him—if you think God is the One who is sending it instead? If Satan can convince you that the Lord wants you sick, then you won't actively fight against it. You may beg and plead for God to set you free, but you won't fight sickness until you know that God isn't its author. If you don't believe that Jesus purchased healing as part of His atonement, then you won't resist infirmity and disease. If you aren't persuaded in your heart that God wants you well, you might ask for deliverance, but you won't actively fight against sickness or stand in faith for healing.

You need to get the same attitude toward sickness that you have toward sin! I'm not condemning you if you get sick any more than I would condemn you if you sin. (Romans 8:1–2.) Christians are redeemed from sin. The power of sin has been broken over us, and we are dead to sin. (Romans 6:11–14.) We should not be living in sin, but there is forgiveness. There is grace if you do sin, so I'm not condemning you. Every born-again believer has had to live with the fact that we haven't lived up to God's standard, and I'm not condemning you for that. Likewise, I'm not condemning a Christian who is sick. However, I am condemning the attitude that says, "Sickness is something God wants for us." That attitude is just as bad as saying, "Sin is something God wants for us." No, that's wrong. Jesus redeemed us from sin, and at the very same time He also redeemed us from sickness.

Now, you can learn something if you go out and sin. You could take drugs, blow out your mind, do stupid things, get in car wrecks, and be arrested. You could get drunk, participate in immorality and perversion, and get a sexually transmitted disease. You can learn from experience that doing these kinds of things is foolish and that there are much better things you could do, but that doesn't mean that God wanted you to get drunk, have a car wreck, and get arrested to teach you that you should be seeking Him more. You could learn through such experiences as those, but did God want you to do that? No. Nobody would say, "God made me get drunk and high, and get arrested, so He could humble me." We wouldn't say that because we recognize that Jesus died to set us free from sin.

Oppressed of the Devil

In the same way that Jesus died to set you free from sin, He also died to set you free from sickness. In the same way that

Christ does not lead you into sin, neither does He bring you infirmity or disease. God is not the author of the sickness that comes against you!

In Acts 10, Peter was preaching the Gospel to Cornelius and his household. He summarized the life and ministry of Jesus, saying:

> *God anointed Jesus of Nazareth with the Holy Ghost and with power: who went about doing good, and healing all that were oppressed of the devil; for God was with him.*
>
> *Acts 10:38*

Notice that the Word says that when Jesus went about healing people it was good. Some churches today think that people who pray for others and claim that they're healed are of the devil. That's contrary to what the Word of God says here in this verse. When Jesus healed the sick, the Bible declares that it was good and it brought glory to God. Things that bring glory to God and draw people closer to Him are not of the devil. Satan is not out healing people.

Jesus went about doing good—healing all who were oppressed of the devil. Notice that they were oppressed of the devil, not of God. God is not the author of sickness, infirmity, or disease.

Prophecy Fulfilled

Isaiah prophesied powerfully of the coming Messiah in chapter 53, saying:

> *He is despised and rejected of men; a man of sorrows, and*

acquainted with grief: and we hid as it were our faces from him; he was despised, and we esteemed him not. Surely he hath borne our griefs, and carried our sorrows: yet we did esteem him stricken, smitten of God, and afflicted. But he was wounded for our transgressions, he was bruised for our iniquities: the chastisement of our peace was upon him; and with his stripes we are healed.

Isaiah 53:3–5

Earlier in my life, I always heard this passage changed and interpreted to say, "This isn't talking about physical healing. It's just speaking of emotional and spiritual healing. In a symbolic sense, we were all cripples limping through life because of the damage sin had done to us. Jesus came to set us free from that." However, if you study the Hebrew meanings of the words in the original language here, especially in verse 4, they clearly refer to physical healing.

In fact, Matthew 8:16–17 describes Jesus actually fulfilling this prophecy from Isaiah 53:4.

When the even was come, they brought unto him many that were possessed with devils: and he cast out the spirits with his word, and healed all that were sick: That it might be fulfilled which was spoken by Esaias [Isaiah] the prophet, saying, Himself took our infirmities, and bare our sicknesses.

Notice how Matthew in the New Testament, quoting Isaiah 53:4 under the inspiration of the Holy Spirit, interpreted griefs and sorrows to mean "infirmities" and "sicknesses." This scripture makes it very clear that Isaiah wasn't speaking of spiritual and emotional healing. Of course, spiritual and emotional healing is included in our salvation benefits, but these verses are speaking specifically about the physical healing of our bodies. The context in Matthew proves this. When Jesus cast these demons out and healed all that were sick, the Bible says this was the fulfillment of Isaiah's prophecy.

In light of Matthew 8:16–17, it's clear that when Isaiah 53:4–5 says that He bore our sorrows and carried our griefs, and that by His stripes we are healed, this is not just referring to some kind of spiritual or emotional healing. It's talking about the physical healing of our bodies. The commentary of Matthew 8 on Isaiah 53 verifies this powerful truth.

Slicing Up the Atonement

We've already looked at many scriptures that clearly reveal physical healing as an important part of Christ's atonement. Since it's part of what Jesus bled, died, and resurrected to provide for us, it's not optional. That's why it's incorrect to say, "Let's not preach healing. Let's just focus on the forgiveness of sins." That's slicing up the atonement into different parts and saying, "Some parts of what Jesus did are important and others aren't." Not true. All of what Jesus did for us—all that He suffered, died, and rose again to provide—is important.

We are not honoring the Lord to pick and choose, and to present a less-than-true picture of the message that He really wants us to communicate. We are not glorifying God by ignoring, neglecting, and/or disbelieving an important part of the full salvation package He has provided. We've made the Gospel message irrelevant to many people because they see it as only applying to the future. They perceive salvation as having no relevance to our present-day situations, which is absolutely incorrect.

Chapter 5

Sickness and Sin

It's always God's will to heal us. We know this because Jesus only did what He saw His Father do.

Then answered Jesus and said unto them, Verily, verily, I say unto you, The Son can do nothing of himself, but what he seeth the Father do: for what things soever he doeth, these also doeth the Son likewise.

John 5:19

God the Son is the express image of God the Father.

Who being the brightness of his glory, and the express image of his person, and upholding all things by the word of his power, when he had by himself purged our sins, sat down on the right hand of the Majesty on high.

Hebrews 1:3

The Greek word translated "express image" speaks of an identical copy or a perfect representation.[1] Therefore, God's Word reveals that Jesus Christ is the identical copy and perfect representation of His Father. He only spoke what He heard His Father say, and He only did what He saw His Father do. So we can be confident in determining God's will concerning healing by looking at the life of Jesus.

Perfect Representation

There is not one example in the Gospels of Jesus ever putting sickness on anyone. The modern church that preaches "God makes people sick" is representing Him completely contrary to the perfect representation of Christ. It's totally opposite of the exact image Jesus gave us of His Father. Not one single time did Jesus ever make anyone sick. Not once did He ever refuse to heal someone. Now, there are a couple of times where people refused to receive healing from Him, but it wasn't because Jesus didn't want to minister it to them. They wouldn't receive it (I'll deal with this more later). There isn't one single time that Jesus said, "No, God wants you sick." He never laid hands on a person and gave him or her an infirmity or a disease. That's not the way Jesus represented God the Father.

There are seventeen times in the Gospels where Jesus healed all of the sick that were present. There are forty-seven other instances where Christ healed at least one or two people at a time (see the section "Is It Always God's Will to Heal?" at the back of this book). But you cannot find even one instance where Jesus refused to heal a person or where He put sickness on someone.

God anointed Jesus of Nazareth with the Holy Ghost and with power: who went about doing good, and healing all that were oppressed of the devil; for God was with him.

Acts 10:38

God is not the author of sickness—He's the author of healing.

Blessing or Curse?

Even under the Old Testament law, sickness, infirmity, and disease were never considered "blessings." Deuteronomy 28:1–14 lists the blessings promised to those who would keep God's commandments, and verses16–68 describe the curses that would come upon those who didn't.

Now, you need to understand that we're in the New Covenant today. We don't have to keep all of the Old Testament law in order to receive the blessings of God. Jesus redeemed us from the curse of the law so that the blessing can come upon us by faith in Him.

> *Christ hath redeemed us from the curse of the law, being made a curse for us: for it is written, Cursed is every one that hangeth on a tree: That the blessing of Abraham might come on the Gentiles through Jesus Christ; that we might receive the promise of the Spirit through faith.*
>
> *Galatians 3:13–14*

Therefore, in Christ we have access by faith to the blessings listed in Deuteronomy 28, and in Christ we have been redeemed and delivered from the curses listed in Deuteronomy 28. However, this chapter of the Bible still shows us what God considers to be "blessings" and "curses."

Imagine a chalkboard with a line drawn down the middle dividing it into two columns. At the top of the left column is the word, "Blessings." At the top of the right column is the word, "Curses." According to Deuteronomy 28, health would be listed

33

on the left in the blessings column, and sickness would be listed on the right in the curses column. Yet many people in the church today reverse this, saying, "Oh, no. It's really a blessing that God gave me this sickness." That's not true.

Roadblocks

Can some good come out of people being sick? Certainly. It's just like the person who learned from the hard knocks of sin. While doing something terribly wrong, they realize, "Man, my life is totally out of balance. I'm a messed up person. I might even be demonized. I need to turn to God!" So they call on the name of the Lord in faith, receive salvation, and get delivered. I've actually talked with individuals who are in prison for murder and are on death row; that's where they decided to turn to the Lord and become born again. Several inmates in this situation have heard my radio programs and written to me. God used what was happening in their lives to bring them to the end of themselves and cause them to become born again. Now their whole life is changed, and they are gloriously saved and serving God. I'm sure you can see that this could happen, but is it correct to say that the Lord caused them to go commit that murder? No, that wasn't God. I can guarantee you that the Lord tried to put restraints on them and obstacles in their way.

God tried to stop those two teenage boys from doing what they did at Columbine High School on April 20, 1999. They killed twelve fellow students, a teacher, and then themselves, while wounding twenty-three others. One of those boys was in a youth Bible study the week before he did that. The minister conducting the Bible study received a word of knowledge from the Lord, interrupted the study, and said, "Somebody here is either thinking about killing themselves or killing someone else." He gave an invitation for a long period of time and pleaded for that person to respond, but he didn't. The very next week this boy and another went out and killed all of those people. God was putting a roadblock in that young man's life. He was dealing with him and trying to turn him from that course of action. It wasn't God that led him to kill people, and then kill himself and send himself to hell. No, God tried to stop him.

There are other individuals who have gone ahead and killed someone, and then at some point afterwards turned to the Lord in repentance and faith. The Lord can use even the things that the devil does in our lives, but that doesn't mean He caused them.

In the same way, Satan has caused people to be sick, infirm, and diseased. Yet, when they get into these terrible situations, they cry out to God, turning wholeheartedly to Him, and He answers their prayers. After being gloriously saved, individuals may learn that they were just self-centered people before. They didn't care about God or anyone else. They may learn important lessons through their infirmity and because of that, mistakenly begin to credit God with giving them that sickness. God would no more give someone sickness to humble them than He would cause them to murder somebody to humble them.

Resist Sickness

Healing is part of Christ's atonement just as much as forgiveness of sins. In the same way that I should resist sin, I should resist sickness. I shouldn't accept infirmity or disease just the same as I wouldn't say, "Well, God. I know that You could help me not to sin, but I don't know if You want me not to sin. Maybe it's Your will for me to sin." Nobody would advocate that type of an attitude, yet modern Christianity does exactly that when it comes to healing. "God, we know You can if it's Your will. We ask You to heal us" and then they just leave it up there. If they get healed, then it must have been God's will. If they don't, then it must not have been.

That's as wrong as a person praying, "God, if You don't want me to go out and commit adultery, then stop me." And if they don't do it, they say, "Thank You, God, for stopping me." But if they do it, then they say, "It must have been God's will for me to commit adultery." We would never say that because adultery is sin. But they see sickness as something that is optional. No, healing is paid for and available just as much as forgiveness of sin. Therefore, we ought to hate sickness and disease as much as we hate sin.

As long as you can tolerate sickness and sin, you will. But once you reach the place of saying, "I'm not living like this, I will not do it; I'll die before I go out and do this," you'll start seeing sin diminished in your life. Once you get the attitude that, "I will not put up with sickness, infirmity, and disease, I resist it in Jesus' name," you'll start seeing healing manifest in your life.

Of course, there's more to it than just this. Among other things, there are laws that govern healing. There's much to learn about receiving healing from God, but this has to be your foundation. Healing is included in Christ's atonement.

God's Will Is Clear

I am seeing a tremendous amount of victory in the area of healing personally and in ministering to others. Unless you are having better results, you ought to consider these truths I'm sharing. This is a foundational truth that makes everything else work: Jesus bore our stripes on His body to heal our bodies just as much as He died to forgive our sins.

Without exception, all the people I've studied who have had the healing power of God manifest in their lives and ministries on a regular basis have had this same foundational belief. I'm not talking about someone who just every once in awhile sees healing. Even an old blind squirrel will come up with a nut every once in awhile. I'm talking about the people who walk in divine health and consistently see miracles of healing. Every single one of them has believed that healing is part of the atonement of the Lord Jesus Christ. They believe it's always God's will to heal just the same as it's always God's will to save.

Until you get that attitude, Satan will always be able to make you passive. Remember, you have to resist—actively fight against—the devil before he'll flee from you. (James 4:7.) You need to understand and believe that healing is from God and sickness is from Satan. Once you make this clear distinction in your heart, then you must resist the devil—and all the sickness, infirmity, and disease he sends your way. You can't just passively say, "Lord, if it's Your will, heal me." You must be persuaded in your heart of the truth of God's Word concerning healing, and then actively stand against the devil.

God's Word is His will, and it's very clear:

Beloved, I wish above all things that thou mayest prosper and be in health, even as thy soul prospereth.

3 John 2

God wants you well!

Chapter 6

A Cop Out

Healing is part of Christ's atonement. It's not a separate issue from salvation. The very Greek word that was used for salvation over a hundred times in the New Testament was also translated healed, made whole, and saved in reference to healing the sick. God never intended for what Jesus accomplished through His death, burial, and resurrection to be broken up and separated into different elements.

Some people have said, "We're going to accept forgiveness of sins, but reject healing, prosperity, and deliverance." No, it's actually all a package deal. It's wrong for the Church to present healing as some fringe benefit that "could happen, but certainly isn't part of our salvation. It's just up to the Lord whether He chooses to heal or not." God's will is to heal you just as much as it is to forgive you. He wants you to resist sickness and disease just as much as He wants you to resist sin.

Part of the Fall

I've often thought about why anybody would fight against healing. Being well seems to be a universal desire. Consider the effort people put into getting their bodies well. They spend untold amounts of money on doctor's visits, medications, and operations. Medications alone are huge in today's society. People are taking these drugs that produce all kinds of side effects. I've seen advertisements on television for different medications that caused so many terrible side effects that I've thought in my heart, *I'd rather be sick than have all of those side effects.* Yet many people will put up with them. They take radiation and chemotherapy that causes their hair to fall out. They'll take drugs that make them swell. People will literally have parts of their bodies cut off in an effort to live. Nobody likes sickness!

Even hypochondriacs don't like it. They may have a fear of sickness that draws them into it and causes them to obsess over it, but they don't like it. People universally hate sickness and disease.

That's because God didn't create mankind to die. Death was something man chose, but it wasn't something God chose. The Lord originally intended for our bodies to live forever. I've actually read some medical reports that say that the body is capable of healing and repairing itself. The medical profession really cannot understand why the body doesn't live forever. Of course, there are these invaders, like germs and viruses, but we have the capacity to overcome them. God's original plan was for us never to be sick. Sickness was not a part of God's plan—it was part of what we unknowingly chose in the Fall.

We were created with a God-given desire on the inside of every one of us for health. People don't like sickness. God doesn't like it. Why then do some people fight against God being our Healer? They'll actually say, "You are of the devil" if you believe that the Lord heals today. Why would somebody argue that when health is a universal need and desire? Everybody wants health. Why would we credit God with wanting something less for our health than the best?

There are also lesser manifestations of this same attitude. These people may not say you're of the devil if you believe for healing. They may not reject you for laying hands on the sick and believing for them to recover. (Mark 16:18.) But they would certainly say, "It's not God's will to heal every single time." Why would they think that? I've already proven earlier in this book that healing is part of the atonement. God provided healing for our bodies just as much—and at the very same time—as He provided forgiveness of sins. With this being so obvious, why do people fight against healing?

A Common Root

Although there are many reasons why people are prejudiced, biased, and teach against healing, I believe they all stem from a common root. People resist the truth that healing is in the atonement and it is God's will to heal every time because it's convenient to believe that way. There may be some sincere people who have been taught wrong, but the bottom line of this teaching against healing is that it's a copout. It avoids the responsibility that becomes ours when we accept that God wants us well.

If the Lord has provided healing for us, and it's obvious that not everybody is healed, then the question arises, "Why aren't we well?" If God wants us well, and we aren't, this means we have to accept some degree of responsibility. I'll deal with this issue later in the book when I discuss why everyone isn't healed, however, for now we need to realize that we must accept some responsibility. In an effort to dodge responsibility and guilt, we often simply say, "Well, it must not have been God's will." That's not true.

Some people argue, "If God wanted someone healed, then they'd be healed whether you or I prayed for them or not." That's not true either. Consider the forgiveness of sins. God's Word says that...

> *The Lord is not slack concerning his promise, as some men count slackness; but is longsuffering to us-ward, not willing that any should perish, but that all should come to repentance.*
> *2 Peter 3:9*

You can't make it any clearer than that. God's will is for people to be saved. Yet, not everybody is saved. Jesus Himself prophesied that more people would choose the broad gate that leads to destruction than the narrow gate that leads to everlasting life.

> *Enter ye in at the strait gate: for wide is the gate, and broad is the way, that leadeth to destruction, and many there be which go in thereat: Because strait is the gate, and narrow is the way, which leadeth unto life, and few there be that find it.*
> *Matthew 7:13–14*

God's will concerning salvation doesn't automatically come to pass. He's not willing that anyone perish, but that all come to repentance and the knowledge of Him. The Lord doesn't will for anyone to die and go to hell, but He gave us a choice. People go to hell because they reject God's provision. Some reject it blatantly in open rebellion against the Lord. Others reject it because they are taught wrong, so they're trusting in their own good works, like attending church, being moral, or tithing. (Romans 10:2–3.) Although they've been deceived, it's still their choices that caused them to miss heaven.

Accept Responsibility

God doesn't want anyone to go to hell, but they do. He doesn't want anyone to be sick either, but they are. Certainly, some people are in total rebellion towards the Lord and His ways, and they're reaping what they've sown. Yet, other people desire healing, and they still fall short. This is because they don't understand how to receive healing properly.

Some people think that being a good person, attending church, and being water baptized as an infant will produce salvation in their life. They may be sincere, but they're sincerely wrong. Although it's not God's will for them to perish, people are perishing. It's not God's will for people to be sick either, but they are. They don't understand how to receive healing.

We need to understand and accept our part. It's our failure, not God's, that sends people to hell and causes us to be sick. It's our failure to accept this responsibility that's the root of why people fight against healing. We do not want to accept responsibility. We don't want to confront the truth that as a believer in Christ we could have done something to prevent that loved one from suffering under sickness and dying.

I'm not saying that it's our fault directly, although in some cases it could be. Often it's not an individual's sin that brought sickness and disease, but mankind's sin that has corrupted this world. It's the sin that caused germs and viruses, fungi and infections, and things like that which were never a part of God's original plan for mankind. They're a perversion of nature that happened through sin, not necessarily individual sin, but the collective sin that has corrupted the entire system. Even though it might not be something we did individually that caused sickness, there is always something we can do individually to overcome that perversion and walk in health.

Not God's Will

Back in the early 1970s, I pastored a church in a small town in Texas. A couple in this church had a child who was born mongoloid. (That's not intended as a slur. I realize that we don't use that term anymore, but that's what these parents called it. I'm just repeating what they said.) The mother was a very small woman, and she and her husband had been living in Guatemala at the time of their son's birth. She delivered this baby boy in a taxi on the way to the hospital and it caused him to have brain damage.

Because he was born mongoloid, his immune system was deficient. The doctor said that if the child ever got a cold, he would die because there was nothing they could do for him. They didn't expect him to live, but he did. When I met them, he was four years old.

Eventually, he did get a cold. So I went to their house and prayed over him to be healed. While holding the child in my arms, he died. We sat there with the parents and prayed for this little boy to be raised from the dead for hours. We did everything I knew to do. Finally, we called the authorities.

The police showed up, and it was a miracle that we didn't all get sent to jail. Really, the only reason they didn't arrest us was because the parents had the medical reports proving that the doctors had said, "If he ever gets sick or has an infection, just keep him at home because there's nothing we can do for him." Since they had those papers, the police let us go. It was a very tragic situation.

The parents asked me to do his funeral. I was groping for something to say that would comfort both them and me. I had taken this personally. It would have been comforting momentarily to have just said, "Well, it couldn't have been us that missed it. We gave it everything we've got." The parents were grieving, and I certainly didn't want to point the finger at them by saying, "It's your fault." It would have been comforting to come up with some of the clichés that you hear commonly given in religion: "God works in mysterious ways. He must have wanted your son in heaven. God needed him there." But I had to be honest with the Word.

So I told those parents, "I don't believe this was God's will. The Lord did not kill your son. He didn't allow this to happen. Satan was the one who snuffed his life out. Even though the devil may have won this battle, he didn't win the war." Then I shared

45

from 2 Samuel 12:23 and other scriptures how this child was now in the presence of God. I ministered hope, and the reality that this boy was with Jesus.

"The Truth Shall Make You Free"

But when it came to why it happened, I basically said, "It's either my fault, your fault, both of our faults, or things that we don't understand. I don't know what it is, but I can guarantee you it's not God." That wasn't as comforting as if I would have said, "Well, God works in mysterious ways. He allowed it. The Lord did this for some reason." That might have given momentary comfort, but the Bible says:

> *Ye shall know the truth, and the truth shall make you free.*
> *John 8:32*

God's Word is true, and I couldn't find in there where Jesus made people sick. I just had to tell them, "I don't know where the problem is, but it's not God. Satan beat us. He won a battle, but he didn't win the war. Your son is now with Jesus, but it wasn't God's will for him to go now due to sickness." Because I told these people the truth, they prayed and God showed them some areas where they had allowed fear, doubt, and unbelief in. This had hindered their faith and kept them from receiving the miracle they needed. Because they received the truth, they repented and were able to overcome that fear.

The doctors had told this woman that the reason her child was mongoloid was because she was so small. They said that the baby should have been taken by a C-section. They concluded that if she ever got pregnant again, the baby would probably have to be taken by C-section, and that both she and the child would probably lose their lives. So they told her never to have another child again.

That was back in the early 1970s. Since then, she's had three or four more children. She recently sent me a picture of all of her kids. They had graduated high school and were in college. She had all natural childbirths at home without any doctor's help because she knew that no doctor after seeing her records would ever allow her to have another baby. So she just believed God. Instead of going childless and living her entire life in bitterness, wondering, *God, why did You do this?* she found out that God wasn't the author of sickness, disease, and death. This precious sister was able to go on and have other children because she took hold of the truth, and the truth set her free.

We Fail to Receive

I understand why people want to say, "Surely this must have been God's will," because it makes us look good. It doesn't make us look like a failure. But it's an easy way out—a cop out. I understand it, and have been tempted to do the same thing, but it's not God who makes people sick. It's not God who fails to heal people; it's us who fail to receive.

My teaching entitled *You've Already Got It!* expands and expounds on these concepts more than I'm able to here. Even though it's applied generally to the Christian life, I give many

47

examples of healing and teaching about healing that prove how God has already healed us. It's not a matter of God giving us healing; it's a matter of us reaching out and by faith receiving healing.

Chapter 7

Paul's Thorn in the Flesh

Any time I minister on physical healing, someone brings up Paul's thorn in the flesh. They say, "God gave Paul a thorn in the flesh. He made him sick. Paul tried to believe the Lord for healing, but wasn't healed. Since Paul was such a great man of God—and the Lord didn't heal him—who are we to think that God will heal us?" This misconception is based on a misinterpretation of Scripture.

The Bible does not say that Paul's thorn in the flesh was sickness. You can listen to people who argue that, but it's not what the Word really says.

Lest I should be exalted above measure through the abundance of the revelations, there was given to me a thorn in the flesh, the messenger of Satan to buffet me, lest I should be exalted above measure. For this thing I besought the Lord thrice, that it might depart from me. And he said unto me, My grace is sufficient for thee: for my strength is made perfect in weakness. Most gladly therefore will I rather glory in my infirmities, that the power of Christ may rest upon me. Therefore I take pleasure in infirmities, in reproaches, in necessities, in persecutions, in distresses for Christ's sake: for when I am weak, then am I strong.

2 Corinthians 12:7–10

In verse 7, Paul made it very clear that this thorn in the flesh was a messenger from Satan, not from God. The Greek word translated "messenger" here is also rendered "angel" elsewhere in the New Testament.[1] (Luke 1:13; 2 Corinthians 11:14; Galatians 4:14, for instance.) Therefore, this was a demonic messenger, a dark angel, sent from the devil to buffet Paul.

From the Devil

Some people erroneously suppose that God gave this thorn in the flesh to Paul because this kept him from being exalted above measure. They just automatically think that this is saying the thorn in the flesh was sent from God to keep him humble. Not true.

Humility is important, but there's also a godly type of exaltation that is mentioned many times in both the Old and New Testament scriptures. One example is 1 Peter 5:6, which says:

> *Humble yourselves therefore under the mighty hand of God, that he may exalt you in due time.*

Being exalted, being lifted up, is good when God does it. However, some people assume that Paul was speaking about pride in 2 Corinthians 12:7. They argue, "Paul had a real problem with pride and arrogance, so God gave him this thorn in the flesh to break him and keep him humble." That's not a godly principle. We just saw that the Bible says to humble yourself. If God humbles you, that's not humility, it's humiliation. Humility is not something you can force on a person. It has to come from the inside out.

Paul's Thorn in the Flesh

Second Corinthians 12:7 is talking about Paul being glorified everywhere he went. He saw people raised from the dead (Acts 20:9–12), demons cast out (Acts 16:16–18), and many other miracles (Acts 19:11–12). The people in one city he ministered at exclaimed, "Those that have turned the world upside down have come here also!" (Acts 17:6.) There was so much power and anointing flowing through Paul's life and ministry that it was drawing many people to the Lord. They were saying, "I want to be like Paul. I want to have the ability to overcome adversity. If I'm thrown in jail for preaching the Gospel, I want an earthquake to come and set me free too!" (Acts 16:25–33.)

Every time something bad happened, Paul saw it turn around for his good. People noticed this, and were saying, "I want that kind of power in my life too!" Satan recognized that Paul was drawing many people to the Lord because he was walking in such absolute victory and being exalted by God. The devil wanted to debase him and do something to keep him from being exalted. That's what 2 Corinthians 12:7 is talking about. Lest Paul be exalted above measure, Satan gave him a thorn in the flesh. It was from the devil, not God.

I've had people who were sick tell me, "I'm like the apostle Paul. God has given me a thorn in the flesh, and I'm just supposed to bear it." Remember, it was because of the abundance of the revelations that this thorn came. With those revelations, Paul wrote half of the New Testament. Therefore, anybody who hasn't had an abundance of revelations like Paul did shouldn't be hiding behind his thorn in the flesh today. Besides, this thorn was from Satan, not God.

When I've tried to start talking to drug addicts, prostitutes, and adulterers about receiving deliverance from God, many of them have told me, "Well, like the apostle Paul, I've just got a thorn in the flesh." They didn't even have a relationship with God, yet they're claiming Paul's thorn in the flesh. If you have been using this thorn-in-the-flesh thing as an excuse, too, you need to quit hiding behind it unless you have so much revelation that you could write half of the New Testament.

Paul's thorn in the flesh was not sickness. It was a demonic messenger sent from Satan to buffet him.

A Weakness or Inadequacy

Another reason some people think Paul's thorn was sickness is that the word "infirmities" is used twice in this passage. Verses 9 and 10 say:

> *And he said unto me, My grace is sufficient for thee: for my strength is made perfect in weakness. Most gladly therefore will I rather glory in my infirmities, that the power of Christ may rest upon me. Therefore I take pleasure in infirmities, in reproaches, in necessities, in persecutions, in distresses for Christ's sake: for when I am weak, then am I strong.*
>
> *2 Corinthians 12:9,10*

This word infirmity is used nearly universally nowadays to refer to some type of a sickness. People say, "This person has an infirmity." We even call the place where we send sick people "the infirmary." Although it has an almost exclusive connotation with sickness in its popular use today, the meaning of this word *infirmity* wasn't limited to sickness at the time that the King James Bible was written. Take, for example, Romans 8:

> *Likewise the Spirit also helpeth our infirmities: for we know not what we should pray for as we ought: but the Spirit itself maketh intercession for us with groanings which cannot be uttered.*
>
> *Romans 8:26*

Notice the colon (:) after the word "infirmities" and again after the word "ought." This verse is saying that it is an infirmity to not know what we should pray for as we ought. If you were to look up the word infirmity in the dictionary, you'd find that it not only means a sickness, but it could also be any weakness or inadequacy. This is how it was used in Romans 8:26. Not knowing how to pray for something is a weakness, an inadequacy, an infirmity—not a sickness or a disease.

Not Sickness

Some people suppose that Paul was talking about sickness here in 2 Corinthians 12:9 when he said, "I...glory in my infirmities." As we look at the context, however, we'll see that it wasn't sickness. We must remember that men put in the chapter and verse divisions later for the purpose of reference. There's nothing wrong with that, but we need to remember that the book we call 2 Corinthians was all one letter. It wasn't broken up by chapter and verse divisions. In what we call 2 Corinthians 11, Paul talked about his infirmities too. He said:

If I must needs glory, I will glory of the things which concern mine infirmities.

2 Corinthians 11:30

Starting in verse 23, Paul defined, explained, and listed what he was calling "infirmities."

Are they ministers of Christ? (I speak as a fool) I am more; in labours more abundant.

2 Corinthians 11:23

As this list continues, keep in mind that these are all the things that just a few verses later Paul summarized by saying, "I'm going to glory in these infirmities." (v. 30; 12:9.) He called "labours more abundant" (hard work), an infirmity. It caused weakness, stress, and problems in his life.

In stripes above measure, in prisons more frequent, in deaths oft. Of the Jews five times received I forty stripes save one.

2 Corinthians 11:23,24

Five times Paul was whipped with thirty-nine stripes.

Thrice was I beaten with rods.

2 Corinthians 11:25

Three times he was cruelly beaten with an instrument similar to a metal rod. This was often done on the feet, resulting in broken bones.

Once was I stoned.

2 Corinthians 11:25

This happened in Acts 14:19. I personally believe he died in that instance.

> *Thrice I suffered shipwreck, a night and a day I have been in the deep; In journeyings often, in perils of waters, in perils of robbers, in perils by mine own countrymen, in perils by the heathen, in perils in the city, in perils in the wilderness, in perils in the sea, in perils among false brethren; In weariness and painfulness, in watchings often, in hunger and thirst, in fastings often, in cold and nakedness. Beside those things that are without, that which cometh upon me daily, the care of all the churches. Who is weak, and I am not weak? who is offended, and I burn not? If I must needs glory, I will glory of the things which concern mine infirmities.*
> *2 Corinthians 11:25–30*

Persecutions and Hardships

All of these things listed were talking about persecution hardships that Paul endured for the cause of Christ. Then, just a few verses later, he declared:

> *Most gladly therefore will I rather glory in my infirmities.*
> *2 Corinthians 12:9*

In context, "infirmities" here is talking about all of the hardships that he suffered for the Gospel. It's a wrong assumption to just take the word *infirmity* and assume that it refers to sickness when, in context, Paul never indicates this is the case. Remember, Romans 8:26 used the same word—"infirmities"—to refer to a lack of knowledge or understanding about how to pray.

55

So we've seen that Paul's thorn in the flesh was a messenger from Satan (2 Corinthians 12:7), and many people jump to the conclusion of sickness because of this word *infirmity*. Yet, in context it was used in a different way here, to describe the persecutions and hardships Paul suffered because of the Gospel. Verse 10 goes on to make this point very clear, saying:

> *Therefore I take pleasure in infirmities, in reproaches, in necessities, in persecutions, in distresses for Christ's sake: for when I am weak, then am I strong.*
>
> *2 Corinthians 12:10*

Although some people assume the word "infirmities" here means physical sickness, the other four things listed in this verse, and the context of 2 Corinthians 11:23–33, reveal otherwise. The other four things listed in 2 Corinthians 12:10 are *reproaches, necessities, persecutions,* and *distresses.* Every one of these makes it very clear that this is not talking about some kind of physical sickness. Rather, it was speaking of a hardship or persecution that Paul had to deal with.

"Reproaches" are insults, injuries, harms, and hurts. "Necessities" refers to doing without certain things for the Gospel's sake. "Persecutions" and "distresses" are easily understood. All of these are consistent with the context of this passage. If Paul was using this word *infirmity* to mean physical sickness, it would be inconsistent with the other things he listed here. His use of the word "infirmities" is referring to the hardships he suffered for the cause of the Lord.

Old Testament Imagery

Furthermore, the people with a Jewish background in the church that Paul was writing to would recognize this phrase "thorn in the flesh" from the early books of the Old Testament.

> *If ye will not drive out the inhabitants of the land from before you; then it shall come to pass, that those which ye let remain of them shall be pricks in your eyes, and thorns in your sides, and shall vex you in the land wherein ye dwell.*
>
> *Numbers 33:55*

Moses told the Israelites that if they did not drive out the inhabitants of the land from before them, then these heathen would persecute and corrupt them. They would be stained and tainted through these pagan people if they let them live.

> *Know for a certainty that the LORD your God will no more drive out any of these nations from before you; but they shall be snares and traps unto you, and scourges in your sides, and thorns in your eyes, until ye perish from off this good land which the LORD your God hath given you.*
>
> *Joshua 23:13*

The Israelites hadn't obeyed God, so the Lord said, "Alright, the prophecy that Moses gave in Numbers 33:55 is going to come to pass." Once again scripture refers to people as being scourges or thorns in their eyes.

> *Wherefore I also said, I will not drive them out from before you; but they shall be as thorns in your sides, and their gods shall be a snare unto you.*
>
> *Judges 2:3*

When Paul used this terminology "thorn in the flesh," the original readers' minds immediately went back to the imagery in the Old Testament scriptures of Numbers 33:55, Joshua 23:13, and Judges 2:3. In each case, it referred to people who were antagonistic toward God's people. This is further biblical evidence that Paul's thorn in the flesh was a demonic personality, a dark angel, a messenger from Satan that stirred up persecutions everywhere Paul went. He made reference to this in his letter to the Corinthians, saying, in essence, "We apostles suffer more than anybody else. The people we minister to are esteemed and blessed, but we are despised and considered the scourges of the earth…"

> *For I think that God hath set forth us the apostles last, as it were appointed to death: for we are made a spectacle unto the world, and to angels, and to men. We are fools for Christ's sake, but ye are wise in Christ; we are weak, but ye are strong; ye are honourable, but we are despised. Even unto this present hour we both hunger, and thirst, and are naked, and are buffeted, and have no certain dwellingplace; And labour, working with our own hands: being reviled, we bless; being persecuted, we suffer it: Being defamed, we entreat: we are made as the filth of the world, and are the offscouring of all things unto this day.*
> *1 Corinthians 4:9–13*

In other words, Paul was talking about the hardships and persecution that he endured. It's apparent in the Word that this demonic messenger worked hard to influence people wherever Paul went, to persecute him. Paul walked in victory, but he also endured more persecution, shipwrecks, beatings, imprisonment, rejection, and criticism than anyone else. Satan used this opposition against him. Even though there was the power of God in manifestation in Paul's life, it was not without a price. This made other people think twice. The devil was doing this to turn people away from Paul's message. They may have even reasoned in their heart, *What he's saying is true, but I'm not sure I'd like to suffer the way he has in order to be able to walk in it.*

"My Grace Is Sufficient"

So Paul sought the Lord three times to remove this thorn in the flesh, this demonic angel that stirred up persecution through people. As we saw in the Old Testament, that's what a thorn in the flesh is: persecution through people. Paul asked Jesus three times to remove it, and the Lord answered:

> *My grace is sufficient for thee: for my strength is made perfect in weakness.*
>
> *2 Corinthians 12:9*

Through Christ's atonement, we have been redeemed from sickness, but not from persecution. Paul himself acknowledged this truth later in his life while writing to Timothy.

> *Yea, and all that will live godly in Christ Jesus shall suffer persecution.*
>
> *2 Timothy 3:12*

Perhaps Paul didn't understand this yet at the time in his life when he asked God to take this thorn in the flesh away. He was pressing in as hard as he could to receive all that the Lord had for him. (Philippians 3:14.) He was even trying to get free from and stop the persecution. Finally, the Lord told him, "Paul, you aren't redeemed from persecution. But I'll give you My grace to deal with it."

Just think, if God had redeemed us from persecution, and He stopped all of our persecutors, there never would have been an Apostle Paul. He himself had been a persecutor. Paul was there participating in the stoning death of Stephen. (Acts 7.) If God would have just wiped out all of the persecutors, there never would have been an Apostle Paul. God doesn't stop all of our persecutors. Rather, He reveals Himself to people through us as we continue to love them, forgive them, turn the other cheek, and follow Jesus. It's a powerful testimony when we continue to love God despite their threats, and God uses it. We aren't redeemed from persecution, but we are redeemed from sickness.

Chapter 8

Eye Problems?

S ome people teach that Paul had a sickness that God refused to heal him of, and therefore we can't expect to be healed of all sicknesses today. That's not true. It's not a consistent interpretation with the whole of God's Word. As we saw in the previous chapter, Paul's thorn in the flesh wasn't sickness, but rather a demonic messenger sent from Satan to stir up persecution.

People who teach that Paul's thorn in the flesh was sickness often misinterpret Galatians 4. Some of them theorize that Paul had some kind of ancient Aramaic eye disease that caused runny, puffy eyes and gave him constant eye problems. They attempt to verify this by this passage.

> *Brethren, I beseech you, be as I am; for I am as ye are: ye have not injured me at all. Ye know how through infirmity of the flesh I preached the gospel unto you at the first. And my temptation which was in my flesh ye despised not, nor rejected; but received me as an angel of God, even as Christ Jesus. Where is then the blessedness ye spake of? for I bear you record, that, if it had been possible, ye would have plucked out your own eyes, and have given them to me.*
>
> *Galatians 4:12–15*

"Infirmity of the Flesh"

Notice the terminology in verse 13, "infirmity of the flesh." This wasn't just an "infirmity," it was an "infirmity of the flesh." He wasn't talking about a lack of understanding (as in not knowing how to pray in Romans 8:26) or a hardship that he endured (like the shipwrecks and perils mentioned in 2 Corinthians 11:25–26). This is literally talking about some kind of a physical problem. Since he used the terminology, "infirmity of the flesh" he qualified it. He basically used this same terminology again in verse 14.

Some people look at this and argue, "Paul said right here that he did have an infirmity!" Yes, he did mention a problem here. But notice what he said in verse 13:

Ye know how through infirmity of the flesh I preached the gospel unto you at the first.

Galatians 4:13

"At the first" implies that it wasn't something long term that God wouldn't heal. It was something temporary. Paul went on to say:

Where is then the blessedness ye spake of? for I bear you record, that, if it had been possible, ye would have plucked out your own eyes, and have given them to me.

Galatians 4:15

Some people say, "Look, now he's talking about an eye problem. That's his infirmity of the flesh." So they theorize that this was a disease of runny, puffy eyes that lasted throughout his entire life. If you can swallow that, then you can make the Bible say anything you want. That is a flimsy basis of interpretation!

Left for Dead

Let's consider a much more accurate interpretation. In order to do so, we need to look at Acts 14. Paul was preaching in Lystra and Derbe. For awhile, the people there thought he was a god.

When the people saw what Paul had done, they lifted up their voices, saying in the speech of Lycaonia, The gods are come down to us in the likeness of men. And they called Barnabas, Jupiter; and Paul, Mercurius, because he was the chief speaker.

Acts 14:11,12

Paul and Barnabas restrained the people from offering a sacrifice and worshiping them. However, the very next day those same people became mad at them.

There came thither certain Jews from Antioch and Iconium, who persuaded the people, and, having stoned Paul, drew him out of the city, supposing he had been dead. Howbeit, as the disciples stood round about him, he rose up, and came into the city: and the next day he departed with Barnabas to Derbe.

Acts 14:19,20

This was an instance where Paul was stoned and left for dead. He refers to this in 2 Corinthians 11:

Once was I stoned.

2 Corinthians 11:25

63

Personally, I believe Paul was dead. If he wasn't dead, he was so close to being dead that the people who were trying to kill him supposed that "he had been dead." (Acts 14:19.) Whether he was dead, or very close to it, the Word says that as the disciples stood round about him, he rose up and came into the city. The next day he departed with Barnabas to Derbe, twenty to fifty miles away (the exact distance is disputed[1]). Paul walked (and/or rode) to the next town, and the following day preached to the people there (vv. 20–21). Can you guess where these cities of Iconium, Lystra, and Derbe were? They were all part of a region called Galatia. These are the people Paul was writing to in Galatians 4 when he said, "At first you took pity on me because of this infirmity in my flesh. You would have plucked out your own eyes for me" (v. 15).

Instead of pulling out of the clear blue sky that Paul had some kind of an ancient eye disease, it's a much more honest interpretation of scripture to recognize that Galatians 4 is referring to the exact same time period where Paul had been stoned, left for dead, rose up, traveled over twenty miles the following day, and began preaching to the people in the next city. Since Paul went from being stoned to death to preaching in the next city in less than twenty-four hours, is it so inconceivable that his eyes might have been hurting him due to the rocks that had repeatedly struck his head the day before?

Although it's obvious that God's miraculous healing power was at work in his body, it probably took Paul some time to fully mend. Paul had said that it was only "at the first" that this "infirmity of the flesh" bothered him (v.13). It's much more accurate to compare scripture with scripture and say that if he did have any eye problems, it was because he had been stoned by some of the city's folks the day before. It was something temporary in his body that healed over time. Paul got over it.

Swallowing a Camel

It's also possible that when Paul said, "You would have plucked out your own eyes and given them to me" that he was using a figure of speech. We say, "You'd give your right arm for me." Does that mean you or I have a bad right arm? No. It's just a figure of speech we use to say that this person would sacrifice anything for me. So Paul saying, "You would have plucked out your own eye and given it to me" may not have had anything to do with him having something wrong with his eyes. If he was talking about the fact that he had some damage to his eyes from the stoning the day before, it was only temporary. He made that very clear in verse 13 by saying, "at the first."

The people who contend that Paul's thorn in the flesh was sickness in the form of some eye disease go on to Galatians 6.

Ye see how large a letter I have written unto you with mine own hand.

Galatians 6:11

I've actually heard someone argue from this that Paul was so nearly blind because of his eyesight problem that his handwriting was three or four inches tall. They said that he had to write huge letters to be able to communicate. If that were true, and Paul was referring to large-size letters, can you imagine how big this letter to the Galatians had to have been? It would have been volumes and volumes. Nobody could have carried it! He would have had only one or two words on a page. Just count how many words there are in Galatians. That's not what Paul was talking about here.

There are different words for talking about size or quantity in the Greek language. The word translated "large" in Galatians 6:11 is the one for quantity.[2] Paul wasn't talking about how big and tall each individual letter of each word was. He was saying, "This letter—this piece of correspondence—that I've written you has become so long." In my Bible, Paul's letter to the Galatians takes up four pages of small print. If you were to print that out in twelve-point type (Times New Roman font), double-spaced on regular sheets of 8.5 x 11 paper, it would be more than eight pages long. I would consider that a large letter, in the sense that it's long. Most personal notes are only a page long, or less.

The people who argue that Paul was saying that every individual letter of each word he wrote was so big are "straining at a gnat and swallowing a camel" (Matthew 23:24 NIV). People who use these scriptures to say that Paul had an eye disease are breaking every rule of sound Bible interpretation. They're just taking a reference and interpreting it any way they want. If Paul did have any eye problems referred to in Galatians 4, it was because he was stoned and left for dead the day before, and it was only temporary. That would be the only correlation between what Paul was saying in Galatians 4 and his mentioning of the thorn in the flesh in 2 Corinthians 12.

Eye Problems?

Paul's thorn in the flesh was not some type of sickness. It was a demonic messenger sent from Satan to stir up persecution wherever he went. We are redeemed from sickness, but not from persecution.

Chapter 9

Redeemed from the Curse

I've given these different interpretations of Paul's thorn much thought, study, and prayer. I've listened to other people and considered their positions. Yet, I believe that what I have shared with you is more honest and more consistent with the whole of Scripture than any other interpretation. Interpreting Paul's thorn in the flesh as sickness is a convenient theology. In other words, it requires no effort on your part. You can just live carnally. You don't have to seek God. You just pray a prayer, and if the person doesn't get healed, you say, "Well, it must be like Paul's thorn in the flesh. God just wants you to bear it." That's a cop out!

The truth is that the Lord wants people healed. But He has to have someone who can operate in faith, use their God-given authority, exercise His power, and make it manifest. This puts responsibility on us, and many of us have become masters at dodging responsibility.

"Don't Drink the Water"

Some people have tried to use 1 Timothy 5 to counter the truth that it's always God's will to heal. Paul was talking to his son in the faith, Timothy, saying:

Drink no longer water, but use a little wine for thy stomach's sake and thine often infirmities.

1 Timothy 5:23

I've actually heard people teach from this that Timothy had some chronic sickness from which he was never healed. Therefore, if Timothy, who was Paul's right-hand man, didn't get healed, then it's not God's will to heal us either.

This is just one verse of scripture. It's the only verse in the entire New Testament that talks about Timothy and taking a little wine for his stomach's sake. There is nothing else to compare this with. Therefore, anything you say about this is supposition, including that he had some chronic sickness. To offer this verse based on that supposition as proof that God doesn't want to heal us is an inaccurate and dishonest interpretation of scripture.

Apparently, whatever sickness Timothy had was a stomach problem, and it was related to the water. What happens when you travel to some third-world country and drink the water? That's right, stomach trouble. In Mexico, they call it Montezuma's Revenge. It's because the water isn't good to drink. Although I haven't personally experienced this, I have seen many people who have traveled with me to other countries get sick drinking the water. I've heard horror stories of how it bothered them. When the water somewhere isn't clean and safe to drink, there are times when it's better to drink something besides water. So Paul was counseling Timothy to quit drinking the water because that's what was causing his stomach problems, and instead to drink a little wine.

This isn't some endorsement for medicine. Some people argue that wine has medicinal qualities and, therefore, Paul was advising Timothy to take medicine for his stomach problems. No, it's very clear that this stomach problem was related to contaminated water. So Paul was saying, "Quit drinking the water and drink wine instead." If they had sodas back then like we do now, he could have said, "Stop drinking the water and have a soda instead." But they didn't have sodas back then, just wine. This is not saying that Timothy had some chronic problem from which he never received healing. This is just Paul telling Timothy, "Quit drinking the water. That's what is causing you to have an upset stomach. Drink something else instead." It's like me speaking to a Bible college student while we're on a mission trip in a foreign country saying, "Don't drink the tap water here. Drink bottled water or have a soda instead, but don't drink the water." That's all he's saying.

From 1 Timothy 5:23, people have invented some kind of a doctrine that makes it look like God wants us to be sick. That's inaccurate. It's not being honest with Scripture.

You Have to Believe

Erastus abode at Corinth: but Trophimus have I left at Miletum sick.

2 Timothy 4:20

Some people argue, "Even one of Paul's companions, Trophimus, didn't get healed. Therefore, it must not be God's will to heal everybody." It's true that not everyone receives healing, but that doesn't mean it's because God doesn't want them to be healed. Not everyone receives salvation, but it's very obvious that God wants everyone to be saved. Just because someone is sick doesn't mean that God willed them to be ill. People infer that because Trophimus was traveling with the apostle Paul, he was a man with faith to be healed. They say, "If it was God's will for him to be healed, he would have received."

People have come up to me in much the same way, if an associate or an employee of mine is ill, has some kind of a sickness or undergoes an operation, or they wear glasses, people will ask, "If it was God's will to heal them, then how come they aren't healed?" I can't manifest healing for another person only on my faith. You don't get healed just by being around someone. It doesn't come by osmosis. You don't rub up against people and receive healing. Each individual has to believe.

Trophimus had to believe. The Word doesn't tell us why he was left at Miletum. Possibly, he was believing, and it just took a period of time for healing to manifest in his body. Yet, Paul didn't want to wait for the manifestation and went on ahead. It's possible that Trophimus was healed and caught up with Paul later on, or ministered in some other way.

It's also possible that Trophimus just quit believing God, so Paul decided to leave him there sick.

There are other possibilities, but there is no reason to interpret Paul leaving Trophimus sick at Miletum as some indication that God doesn't want us to be healed.

Never a Blessing

If we're honest with the Scripture, we've debunked the misinterpretations people use to undermine healing. It's not true to say that God wants certain people sick. You may still be wondering about some scriptures like Romans 8:28, which says that God works all things together for good. I encourage you to check out my teaching entitled, *"The Sovereignty of God."* I've dealt with that verse (and others) there more thoroughly than I can here.

Because of a wrong understanding of God's sovereignty, some people think that the Lord controls everything, and that a person couldn't be sick unless God allowed it. That is not what the Word teaches. Again, God doesn't allow people to go to hell. In one sense, you could say that He allows it because of His high regard for our free will. But it's not His desire, wish, or plan. God puts roadblocks in our way, inviting us to repent and be born again, but ultimately He gives us the choice. God doesn't control us like pawns in a chess game. Anyone who goes to hell has to climb over mountains of obstacles the Lord placed in their path.

Although there are several Old Testament references to where God struck people with sickness, not once was it ever considered a blessing. Both Miriam (Numbers 12) and King Uzziah (2 Chronicles 26) became leprous. A plague killed 185,000 people. (2 Kings 19.) The angel of the Lord went through and killed all the firstborn of the Egyptians in one night. (Exodus 12.) Yes, God put sickness on people under the Old Covenant, but it was never a blessing.

Prior to being struck with leprosy, Miriam had been a great leader among the children of Israel. After this incident, the only thing said about her in the Word was that she died and the people mourned for her. Her ministry was over. The leprosy was a punishment and a curse, not a blessing.

Uzziah had been a king that was mightily used of God. But after being struck with leprosy, it was as if the anointing lifted. He just suffered the whole time. Sickness was a curse, not a blessing. It didn't help him. It hurt him.

The 185,000 people killed by the death angel weren't benefited. It didn't do them any good. It may have made an example out of them, but it wasn't a blessing for them.

In the New Covenant

Deuteronomy 28 states very clearly that sickness is a curse—not good—and health is a blessing. There were times that God smote people with curses, but Galatians 3 reveals that:

> *Christ hath redeemed us from the curse of the law, being made a curse for us: for it is written, Cursed is every one that hangeth on a tree: That the blessing of Abraham might come on the Gentiles through Jesus Christ; that we might receive the promise of the Spirit through faith.*
>
> *Galatians 3:13,14*

Redeemed from the Curse

Christ redeemed us from the curse. Yes, there are instances where God smote people with sickness, leprosy, disease, blindness, and death (2 Kings 1), but it was never a blessing. (Luke 9:54–56.) It was always punishment, and it was always a curse. And in the New Covenant, we are redeemed from the curse.

God's System

Some people wonder, "Well, if God doesn't chastise us with sickness and correct us with tragedy, then how will we learn?" The Bible says:

> *All scripture is given by inspiration of God, and is profitable for doctrine, for reproof, for correction, for instruction in righteousness: That the man of God may be perfect, throughly furnished unto all good works.*
>
> *2 Timothy 3:16,17*

God reproves, corrects, and instructs us through His Word. The Lord's system of correction is not sickness, disease, and tragedy. God disciplines and trains us through His Word. Notice how this verse says the correction of the Word will make you perfect, "throughly furnished unto all good works." That means it's sufficient. You don't need some other form of correction.

Some folks argue, "Yeah, but not everyone obeys the Word. Some people only respond when everything in their life goes sour." Tragedy, sickness, and disease are not God's system. His system is to teach you through the Word—through the Holy Spirit quickening the Word to you. You can learn in other ways, but that's not God's system.

There's no doubt that certain people have become paraplegics, and because of that they've learned to turn to God. He has sustained them, and they walk in much joy and peace, blessing and ministering to many people today. That's good, but it's wrong for them to say, "God made me paraplegic so that I could learn this." No, the Lord tried to teach them by the Holy Spirit through the Word of God.

If you don't respond to the Lord through His Word, there are other ways you can learn. You can learn by hard knocks, if you live through them. Difficult life experiences make exciting testimonies, if you survive them. Many people don't. But that's not God's system. He teaches us through His Word.

Consider These Truths

God can work anything that happens to us together for good, but not everything that happens to us comes from God. (Romans 8:28; John 10:10.) Sickness is not from God. (James 1:16–17.) The Lord doesn't put sickness on you to humble you. God wants you well!

Paul was not afflicted by God. It was a messenger of Satan that came against him. The Lord didn't refuse to heal him, saying, "Just bear it." No, the Lord told him, "Paul, I'll give you grace to endure all the hardship and persecution that the devil and people throw your way." God loved those people. He didn't want to just kill them and wipe them out in order to end all of Paul's problems. There were other Sauls[1] out there who needed to be converted and made spokesmen for God. Therefore, the

76

Lord didn't stop the persecution against the apostle Paul. It was a demonic messenger that stirred up hardship and persecution against him. This thorn in the flesh had been sent by Satan to try to beat Paul down and keep him from being exalted and used of God.

These are powerful truths that are clearly consistent with the whole of God's Word.

It's not God's will for you to be sick, so quit hiding behind Paul's thorn in the flesh. Stop holding on to this religious bias against healing. Turn from this wrong concept that the Lord is putting sickness on you to teach you something today. You need to approach God's Word simply, and honestly consider these truths we've discussed thus far. Look in the Bible for yourself. Consider the context and the meanings of the words in their original languages. As you study for yourself, I believe you'll find what I've shared with you proven true.

It's a religious bias, prejudice, and predetermination that argues that God wants you to be sick. It's a convenient theology that dodges responsibility. Because this bias exists, people have gone to the Word of God and tried to make it say things it doesn't say.

These truths I've shared will help you establish in your heart that it's always God's will for you to be well.

Chapter 10

Jesus Healed Them All

Healing is part of Christ's atonement. (Isaiah 53:4–5.) Therefore it's not an add-on or in addition to salvation. It's a done deal. (1 Peter 2:24.) Through Christ's death, burial, and resurrection, healing has already been provided. Paul's thorn in the flesh was a demonic messenger that stirred up persecution. (2 Corinthians 12:7.) It wasn't sickness. The Lord isn't putting sickness or disease on anyone today. Under the New Covenant, we've been redeemed from the curse of the law. (Deuteronomy 28:15–68; Galatians 3:13–14.) Through faith in Christ and what He's done, every blessing—including health—is now ours in Him. (Deuteronomy 28:1–14; Eph. 1:3.) Hopefully you've already come into agreement with the Word.

If Satan can get you to believe that God wants you sick, that there is some purpose in you being ill, that the Lord is using it for some reason, then it is impossible for you to truly fight against it lest you fight against God. So it renders you passive.

James 4:7 says:

Submit yourselves therefore to God. Resist the devil, and he will flee from you.

We must resist the devil. Resist means "to actively fight against." If Satan can get us into a passive position where we are just saying, "Well, whatever God wills," and we aren't actively fighting against the devil, then he can overcome us with sickness and disease. We need to know that when we are fighting sickness that we are doing God's will and that we aren't fighting against Him or being rebellious toward some type of correction or punishment that He's sent into our life. Basically, religion today has said that sickness comes from God, that He uses it to work His will in our life, and that it's wrong to believe for healing. This has to be totally eradicated from our hearts and minds before we can truly believe and receive our healing. These are the foundations.

Now, once that's established and someone really believes, that doesn't mean that they're just automatically going to be healed. You do have to believe that it's God's will, but then there are other factors that are involved in seeing healing manifest. That's what we are going to look into in these next few chapters. If it is God's will to heal, and if He's not the One who put sickness on us, then why isn't every person healed?

Jesus Hasn't Changed

First of all, when Jesus was here on this earth every person who would allow Him to minister to them was healed. Jesus healed them all, and He didn't do that just once. He did it on a number of occasions. Jesus was the express image of the Father. He said, "I do always those things which I see my Father do." The very fact that Jesus healed all, never refusing to heal a single person, never putting sickness on anyone should be proof enough that God is not the author of our sickness.

Jesus Healed Them All

In the Gospels alone, there are seventeen times where Jesus healed all of the sick that were present. Although Mark, Luke, and John all have examples of this as well, let's look at this truth through the book of Matthew. Jesus did heal them all, and He hasn't changed.

> *Jesus Christ the same yesterday, and to day, and for ever.*
> *Hebrews 13:8*

Christ isn't the One who has changed, His followers have. We aren't representing Him the way He really wants to be represented. It's not God who isn't healing the sick today, it's His followers. We've really fallen in this area.

Matthew 4:23–24 says that:

> *Jesus went about all Galilee, teaching in their synagogues, and preaching the gospel of the kingdom, and healing all manner of sickness and all manner of disease among the people. And his fame went throughout all Syria: and they brought unto him all sick people that were taken with divers diseases and torments, and those which were possessed with devils, and those which were lunatic, and those that had the palsy; and he healed them.*

People with all kinds of sicknesses, diseases, and torments were brought to Jesus and He healed them. He didn't just heal some, He healed them all!

Every Sickness and Every Disease

> *When the even was come, they brought unto him many that were possessed with devils: and he cast out the spirits with his*

word, and healed all that were sick: That it might be fulfilled which was spoken by Esaias the prophet, saying, Himself took our infirmities, and bare our sicknesses.

Matthew 8:16,17

This verse states very clearly that Jesus healed all that were sick—not some of them, but all of them.

Jesus went about all the cities and villages, teaching in their synagogues, and preaching the gospel of the kingdom, and healing every sickness and every disease among the people.

Matthew 9:35

What a powerful statement! Jesus was healing every sickness and every disease among the people. He didn't just have a few people who received, and then others who went away still sick. Jesus healed them all.

But when Jesus knew it, he withdrew himself from thence: and great multitudes followed him, and he healed them all.

Matthew 12:15

Even with great multitudes, He healed them all. It is God's will for you to be well! The life and example of Jesus is clear: He healed them all. The Lord never refused to heal a single person. There were some who refused to receive healing, which I'll deal with later, but He healed all who would receive His ministry.

Jesus went forth, and saw a great multitude, and was moved with compassion toward them, and he healed their sick.

Matthew 14:14

When they were gone over, they came into the land of Gennesaret. And when the men of that place had knowledge of him, they sent out into all that country round about, and brought unto him all that were diseased; And besought him that they might only touch the hem of his garment: and as many as touched were made perfectly whole.

Matthew 14:34–36

Glory to God, Not the Devil

Great multitudes came unto him, having with them those that were lame, blind, dumb, maimed, and many others, and cast them down at Jesus' feet; and he healed them.

Matthew 15:30

Again, this implies that He healed every single one of them. Verse 31 shows the results:

Insomuch that the multitude wondered, when they saw the dumb to speak, the maimed to be whole, the lame to walk, and the blind to see: and they glorified the God of Israel.

Something that brings glory to God is not of the devil. People saying that people being miraculously healed is of the devil is nothing but a cop out. It's an excuse for their powerlessness. It's a way to justify themselves, and to do it they have to condemn those who are following the example of Jesus.

Great multitudes followed him; and he healed them there.

Matthew 19:2

The blind and the lame came to him in the temple; and he healed them.

Matthew 21:14

These are just a few of the seventeen separate examples in the Gospels where Jesus healed all that came to him (the rest are listed at the end of this book in the section called "Is It Always God's Will to Heal?"). Since Jesus said that He did exactly what He saw His Father do, and Hebrews 1:3 says that Jesus was the express image of the Father, this shows that it is God's will to heal us all.

Then why don't we see every single person healed? That's a simple question, but it has a complex answer, which we're going to spend the next few chapters dealing with.

Chapter 11

Why Isn't Everyone Healed?

I f it's God's will to heal us all, then why isn't everyone healed? Jesus' disciples basically asked Him the exact same question in Matthew 17.

> *Then came the disciples to Jesus apart, and said, Why could not we cast him out?*
> *Matthew 17:19*

In the first part of this chapter, Jesus had taken three of His disciples—Peter, James, and John—and gone up onto a mountain. This was where He was transfigured. He literally began to radiate the light of the shekinah glory of God. A cloud overshadowed Jesus and these three disciples, and an audible voice came out of the cloud saying:

> *This is my beloved Son, in whom I am well pleased; hear ye him.*
> *Matthew 17:5*

Elijah and Moses appeared and spoke with Jesus about His crucifixion, which was coming up shortly. These disciples saw all this, and had a miraculous, glorious time. Then they came down from the mountain to the rest of the disciples and the crowd that had gathered there.

When they were come to the multitude, there came to him a certain man, kneeling down to him, and saying, Lord, have mercy on my son: for he is lunatic, and sore vexed: for ofttimes he falleth into the fire, and oft into the water. And I brought him to thy disciples, and they could not cure him.

Matthew 17:14–16

While Jesus was on the mountain with Peter, James, and John, the rest of the disciples were down below. A man had a boy whom the scripture says was lunatic. He suffered from seizures, probably something like epilepsy. This is described in Mark's account of this same instance. (Mark 9:17–29.) So the father brought this boy to Jesus' disciples to cast this demon out, but they couldn't do it.

Then Jesus answered and said, O faithless and perverse generation, how long shall I be with you? how long shall I suffer you? bring him hither to me.

Matthew 17:17

Jesus wasn't pleased with His disciples' inability to effect this healing. If the Lord had been there, He would have healed this boy, and later on He did. Jesus wasn't at all pleased with His disciples' inability to deal with this situation. This is a completely different attitude than what most people have today.

"I've Failed"

As a matter of fact, some people will be critical of my teaching in this book because I'm saying that it's God's will to heal everyone all the time. One of the obvious reasons why we don't see people healed today is that we aren't believing God for it. We are operating in unbelief. Rather than accept that, some folks will criticize me, saying, "You aren't being compassionate. You're just criticizing people you ought to be compassionate towards. You should tell them that they're doing the best they can, and that's fine."

Well, how did Jesus respond? When He found out that His disciples couldn't deal with this situation, He declared, "O faithless and perverse generation! How long shall I be with you? How long shall I put up with you? Bring him here to Me." Do you really think that Jesus would have a more compassionate response to us today? Do you think that the Lord has changed, and now He doesn't want us to minister healing to people? Absolutely not!

I've failed. I don't see healing always come to pass. I've seen some people very close to me die, family and friends I loved with all of my heart. I've had to accept partial responsibility. It's a complex issue. I'm not saying that it was all my fault, all their fault, or all anybody's fault. We're still learning. But I am saying that I know it was God's will for these people to be healed.

I saw my dad die after praying for him for several months to get well. I was only twelve years old at the time. A few years later, I saw a girl I was unofficially engaged to die. (I wasn't really engaged to her, but we had thought about it. I was a soldier in Vietnam and her family told people I was engaged to her, which allowed me emergency leave to come home during that time.) I remember being with her as she passed away. We stood there for hours praying and believing for her to be raised from the dead.

I understand people wanting to dodge responsibility because they just can't cope. If they think that there was something they could have done to have stopped this, then it would make them feel so guilty. They'd have to say, "I've failed." Well, I believe I did fail. I believe that not only me, but this girl, my father, and others—we didn't appropriate what Jesus had provided for us. So yes, we were wrong. But am I condemned by that? No, I'm not condemned at all. I believe that God loves me. He has comforted me. But knowing the truth has motivated me to get in and learn what His Word says and not allow it to happen again. Believe me, I am motivated! I realize it's not God who is letting people die. It's us, and it's because of our unbelief.

We Are Responsible

Jesus said, "You faithless and perverse generation." When people come to the church today with a financial problem, we send them to the lenders saying, "Have you been to the bank? Have you checked in with the social workers?" If they're sick we ask, "Have you been to the doctor? Does he need to operate? Have you taken medication?" If they are depressed and discouraged, we ask "Have you taken any medicine for this? Have you gone to a psychiatrist? You need a shrink and some therapy." In other words, the Church has basically abdicated our authority and responsibility for meeting the needs of people. Today people feel like you are inconsiderate and uncompassionate if you tell people, "We are responsible to minister to the sick, the poor, and the demonized."

Why Isn't Everyone Healed?

Jesus wasn't pleased that His disciples couldn't effect this cure. The Lord is not pleased today that His disciples aren't seeing all of the sick healed. It's God's will to heal every single person every single time. The reason this doesn't happen isn't because God fails to do it. It's because His representatives aren't operating in the fullness of what He's provided for us.

Yes, this puts responsibility on me. Yes, it means that I've missed it. Yes, this means that other people have missed it too. I'd rather maintain God's integrity than my own. God is a good God, and He isn't causing people to die. God is not the One who is putting terminal diseases on people like cancer and AIDS. That's not the way that it is.

Sin

There are three main reasons why people get sick. One of them is sin.

After healing the man at the pool of Bethesda, Jesus said to him:

> *Behold, thou art made whole: sin no more, lest a worse thing come unto thee.*
>
> *John 5:14*

Jesus made it very clear in this verse that this man's sickness returning, and even something worse than what he'd had, could come on him if he sinned. Therefore, Jesus linked sickness with sin. Now, this isn't the only reason that people get sick, but it is one reason.

When alcoholics drink all of their lives and get a liver disease, they did that to themselves. Satan used their actions to gain access to them. They have a liver disease not because God did it, not because the devil did it directly, but because they're reaping the results of their sin. (Romans 6:21–23.) Drug abusers get brain damage. They often contract diseases that are transmitted through shared needles. Sexually promiscuous people get sexually transmitted diseases. This isn't happening because Satan is oppressing them. They're doing it to themselves. They've opened up a door through sin.

A Direct Attack

The second major reason that people get sick is because we are in a battle with the devil. Some people aren't aware of this, but not everything that goes on is merely physical. There is a spiritual battle raging with godly angels carrying out the Lord's will and demonic spirits carrying out Satan's will. Sometimes our enemy just fights us, and it's not based on an individual sin that we do. In a sense, it is sin-based because Satan was loosed into this earth through sin, but the sickness isn't necessarily from your individual sin.

Jesus spoke of this as He walked by a man who had been born blind.

> *His disciples asked him, saying, Master, who did sin, this man, or his parents, that he was born blind? Jesus answered, Neither hath this man sinned, nor his parents: but that the works of God should be made manifest in him.*
>
> *John 9:2,3*

The Lord wasn't saying that neither this man nor his parents had never sinned. The Bible is clear about this point.

All have sinned, and come short of the glory of God.

Romans 3:23

Even though they had sin in their life, Jesus was saying that neither this man's nor his parents' sin had caused this blindness. It just happened. There is a spiritual battle going on, and Satan is going about seeking whom he may devour. (1 Peter 5:8.)

Sin is one reason people get sick. Another reason is that we're living in a fallen world, and there are spiritual battles. Sometimes Satan just attacks us with things. An illness could be nothing but a direct attack from the devil.

Natural Things

The third main reason that people get sick is simply natural things. This is something that many Spirit-filled Christians haven't really taken into account. They recognize the first two reasons—that sin is an inroad of Satan into our lives allowing him to do things, and that we're in a spiritual battle and sometimes the devil just fights us. However, Spirit-filled Christians will often so spiritualize everything that they don't recognize that there are just some things that happen naturally.

If you aren't paying attention while walking down stairs, you could trip, fall, and break your leg, neck, or collarbone. You could have all kinds of negative things happen. Yet, it's not sin or the devil that caused it, it was just something natural. You could hurt

91

yourself, catch a cold, get an infection, have swelling—all kinds of things—for purely natural reasons.

I've heard of people who dove off a cliff, hit a rock in a pool of water, and broke their spine. Now they're quadriplegic. It wasn't necessarily the devil who did that to them. He may have enticed them to go against their better judgment and do something that wasn't wise, but it was natural. When someone loses a limb due to a car wreck, it's not so much the devil, but something natural.

Since mankind fell and sin tainted the earth, all kinds of things like germs, bacteria, viruses, and fungi that were good became corrupted and now fight against our human bodies. In this fallen world, some things are just natural.

One time, a man I knew had an accident while putting a roof on a house. He hit a nail, it broke, then ricocheted off the roof and stuck in his eye. Many people would say, "Well, that's the devil," but mistakes happen. People aren't perfect. Sometimes things are just natural.

There's Always Something We Can Do About It

You can give an inroad to sickness through sin.

It could be natural. When you fall off your house, you're going to hurt yourself. You might hurt something or break something. It's not necessarily demonic. It's not sin. It's just natural. Sometimes stuff like that just happens.

Why Isn't Everyone Healed?

Or the devil could be attacking you through no fault of your own. In fact, when Satan fights against you it's a very good sign that you're doing something right. The enemy seeks to hinder people who are responsive to God and fighting him. You can tell you've arrived at the Promised Land when you meet the giants. When problems are staring you in the face, sometimes it's an indication that you're doing things right instead of wrong.

The good news is that no matter what caused the sickness—sin, the devil, or something natural—there's always something we can do about it. Since the Lord has redeemed us from sickness and disease, we can take our authority, exercise our faith, and effect a cure. Even if our own sin opened a door and brought the sickness on us, we can repent and turn from it, and release the forgiveness and healing power of God in our lives. Regardless of how these sicknesses and diseases come, there's always something we as believers can do about it.

Chapter 12

"Because of Your Unbelief"

A fter Jesus rebuked His disciples, He turned and healed the demonized boy.

Jesus rebuked the devil; and he departed out of him: and the child was cured from that very hour.

Matthew 17:18

The disciples immediately pulled Jesus aside and asked:

Why could not we cast him out?

Matthew 17:19

This is the question we're dealing with. If it's God's will to heal, and Jesus healed this boy, why didn't the disciples see him healed? If we believe that it's God's will for everyone to be healed, then why don't we always see every person healed? What are the reasons why someone isn't healed?

Why They Were Confused

The disciples who asked Jesus this question, "Why could not we cast him out?" believed that it was God's will to heal. They knew they had the power to cast these demons out. They had already been given power and authority to heal the sick and cast out devils. The Bible reveals that seven chapters earlier:

> *When he had called unto him his twelve disciples, he gave them power against unclean spirits, to cast them out, and to heal all manner of sickness and all manner of disease...Heal the sick, cleanse the lepers, raise the dead, cast out devils.*
>
> *Matthew 10:1,8*

The parallel accounts of this passage record that these disciples...

> *Cast out many devils, and anointed with oil many that were sick, and healed them.*
>
> *Mark 6:13*

> *And they departed, and went through the towns, preaching the gospel, and healing every where.*
>
> *Luke 9:6*

Upon their return, there isn't a single question recorded. This means that these same disciples who were asking, "Why couldn't we cast this demon out?" in Matthew 17 had already believed and successfully exercised this power and authority in Mark 6. It wasn't because they didn't believe that they asked this question. They did believe. They had already exercised that power and seen the desired results. This is why they were confused.

If these disciples had thought, *We just don't believe that you can heal a person with this ailment. We don't believe God can do that,* they wouldn't have asked this question. The very fact that they asked this question shows that they did believe, and yet they didn't get the results they desired.

Simple, but Profound

This is important. People who don't believe that God wants us well don't spend much time wondering, *Why isn't everyone healed?* That's because they don't believe it is God's will to heal everyone. The people who are perplexed are those who do believe it's God's will, and yet aren't seeing every single person—perhaps even themselves—healed. Why does that happen?

The answer Jesus gave the disciples to their question of why they couldn't cast the demon out of the boy is very revealing:

Because of your unbelief.

Matthew 17:20

This is simple, but it's profound: "Because of your unbelief."

This is different than what most people would say. If I hadn't led up to this by taking you through this particular passage of scripture, you probably wouldn't have answered what Jesus did. If I had just been talking to you personally and asked, "Why isn't everyone healed?" you probably would have said something like, "Well, they just don't have enough faith." That's the typical answer most people would say.

Now, it's true that if a person doesn't have faith then that will affect their receiving healing. In every instance where Jesus ministered healing, some degree of faith was involved. Some people may argue, "What about in Luke 7:11–16 where Jesus raised the boy from the dead in the city of Nain?" It was faith for this widow mother to allow Jesus to interrupt the funeral procession and her grief. She then responded positively to His command, "Weep not" (v. 13). If faith wasn't present, she and the others there would have reacted very differently. In every instance that Jesus ministered healing, somebody there had to be to some degree in faith.

Reach Out and Take

Sometimes people came to Jesus like the woman in Mark 5:

For she said, If I may touch but his clothes, I shall be whole.

Mark 5:28

She touched the hem of His garment in faith, the power of God flowed, and this woman was healed. The Lord told her, "Your faith has made you whole" (v. 34). Now that's a strong faith. That's a faith that reaches out and takes what God has available.

Not everyone who received healing exhibited that type of faith, but they had to have at least what I call a "passive" faith. You may not have the faith that reaches out and takes it, but if you are going to receive healing off of my prayer and faith, then you must have at least a passive faith that will receive healing if I will bring it to you. This needs further explanation.

We just saw that if you were to ask the average person "Why isn't everyone healed," most people would answer, "Well, it's because they don't have enough faith." It's true that if a person isn't operating in faith it will hinder them from receiving, but that's not what the Lord said.

Jesus said unto them, Because of your unbelief.
Matthew 17:20

He didn't say that it was because they had little faith. He said it was because they had unbelief.

Believe and Disbelieve

Now, certain versions of the Bible render this verse inaccurately saying, "Because you have so little faith." That's a terrible translation! It's not what this verse says. If you were to look in the majority of the translations, especially the more literal ones, this verse is rendered "Because of your unbelief," not "Because you have so little faith."

You may be wondering, *Well, what's the difference? If you have unbelief, then that means you don't have faith. If you have faith, you won't have any unbelief.* No, that's not true.

Most people have this concept that if you are believing God, then that automatically means you don't have any unbelief. If you did have any unbelief, then that automatically means that you don't have any faith. If you were truly in faith, there would be zero unbelief. This is not what the Word teaches.

For verily I say unto you, That whosoever shall say unto
this mountain, Be thou removed, and be thou cast into the
sea; and shall not doubt in his heart, but shall believe that

those things which he saith shall come to pass; he shall have whatsoever he saith.

Mark 11:23

Jesus said you have to speak to this mountain. It's understood that you must speak in faith, and not doubt in your heart. If being in faith truly meant that you automatically had zero unbelief, why then did Jesus include this part about not doubting in your heart? The truth is, you can believe and disbelieve at the same time.

At the Same Time

Consider the parallel passage of this father and his demonized boy in Mark 9:

And they brought him unto [Jesus]: and when he saw him, straightway the spirit tare him; and he fell on the ground, and wallowed foaming. And he asked his father, How long is it ago since this came unto him? And he said, Of a child. And ofttimes it hath cast him into the fire, and into the waters, to destroy him: but if thou canst do any thing, have compassion on us, and help us. Jesus said unto him, If thou canst believe, all things are possible to him that believeth.

Mark 9:20–23

In other words, as the father saw the manifestation of this boy having a seizure, he felt exasperated and frustrated. Finally, he looked at Jesus and said, "If you can do anything, help us." He began to doubt and despair. He was looking at the situation and saying, "God, I don't know if You can even handle this." Instead of accepting all of the responsibility for this healing on

Himself, Jesus turned back to this father and declared, "If you can believe, all things are possible to him that believes."

Now look at how this father responded.

And straightway the father of the child cried out, and said with tears, Lord, I believe; help thou mine unbelief.

Mark 9:24

Jesus didn't say, "Well, that's a stupid statement. If you truly believe, you can't have unbelief. If you have any unbelief, then you aren't really believing." The Lord didn't correct him, rebuke him, or say anything like that. He just turned around and cured the boy. This shows that you can have faith, and yet have unbelief, at the same time.

Faith Canceled Out

Imagine a team of horses hooked up to a wagon. Under normal circumstances, they would have enough power and be able to move that wagon. But if you hooked an equal team of horses up to the other side of the wagon, and had them pulling at the same time in the opposite direction, the net effect would be zero. With both teams of horses pulling on that wagon with all their strength, it wouldn't move because they're canceling each other out. One team is negating the other. They're counterbalancing each other.

This is what Jesus was saying here in Matthew 17:20. He didn't tell His disciples, "It's because you don't have enough faith." He said, "It's because of your unbelief. Your unbelief canceled out the faith you had."

These guys had been in faith before. They had seen demons cast out, and people healed and set free. This time they did the same thing as before, but didn't get the same results. That's why they were confused. They knew they were believing God. So they asked Him, "Why could we not cast him out?" Jesus didn't answer, "Because of your little faith." He said, "It's because of your unbelief."

A Tiny, Little Mustard Seed

Translating this "Because you have so little faith" makes no sense when you look at the rest of the verse.

Jesus said unto them, Because of your unbelief: for verily I say unto you, If ye have faith as a grain of mustard seed, ye shall say unto this mountain, Remove hence to yonder place; and it shall remove; and nothing shall be impossible unto you.
Matthew 17:20

Jesus was saying, "If your faith is only the size of a mustard seed, nothing would be impossible to you." A mustard seed is one of the tiniest seeds there is. It's like one of those poppy seeds on a bun. The point our Lord was making is that even if your faith is tiny, it's enough to cast a mountain into the sea. You don't need big faith, you just need a faith that isn't canceled out, counterbalanced, or negated by unbelief pulling in the opposite direction. Faith the size of a tiny little mustard seed is all you need to speak to a mountain and see it cast into the sea without even physically having to touch it.

If Jesus had really been saying, "It's because you have so little faith," then He would have contradicted and counteracted the very point He was making in the rest of the verse with faith the size of a mustard seed making a mountain move. Do you see how that doesn't fit? It doesn't make sense. Jesus was saying, "Guys, it's not that you didn't believe. It's that your unbelief negated your faith. That's why you didn't see the desired results."

Chapter 13

Faith Negated

Not long after the first time I saw a person raised from the dead, I was excited. I was pumped. I thought, *If I can see someone raised from the dead, then I can see blind eyes opened, deaf ears healed, people come out of wheelchairs—anything!* I was holding a service in Omaha, Nebraska. On my left, in the front, was a man sitting in a wheelchair. I was so excited. I thought, God, I've seen You raise someone from the dead, so I know this guy is going to be healed. I could hardly wait to get through preaching so I could go over and minister to this fellow.

As soon as I finished my message, I went over to him, grabbed him by the hand, and declared, "In the name of Jesus Christ of Nazareth, rise up and walk!" When I yanked him out of the wheelchair, he came up, over, and then fell flat on his face. Since he was paralyzed, he couldn't stand up or catch himself.

When that happened, you could hear the gasps and groans of unbelief and shock from the people. I was shocked. I felt embarrassed and humiliated. I thought, *Look what I've done to this man. I've embarrassed and humiliated him.* It felt terrible. So I got down on my hands and knees, grabbed this guy around his chest, wrestled him back into the wheelchair, and said the equivalent of, "Depart in peace, be ye warmed and filled" (James 2:16). Yet, I didn't give him what he needed. This man left in his wheelchair.

When I returned to the hotel room, I remember asking, "God, why did that happen?" What confused me was the fact that I knew I had faith. Some people may think, *No, if you had faith, he would have been healed.* No, I had faith. I used my faith as far as I could tell, just the same as I did on that man who was raised from the dead. I had just as much faith. It wasn't that I wasn't believing God. You don't go up, grab someone, and pull them out of their wheelchair unless you believe they're going to walk. I didn't expect that man to fall on his face. I expected him to walk. There was faith present, and because I had faith I was confused. Why didn't I see the right results?

Fear of Man

So I asked God, "Why wasn't this man healed?" It took me about three years for my lightning-fast mind to finally figure this out. The Lord showed me, "Andrew, you did have faith, but you also had unbelief." When the people responded in shock and I panicked, that was unbelief. I was more concerned about what other people said than I was about what God had to say.

Jesus said:

> *How can ye believe, which receive honour one of another, and seek not the honour that cometh from God only?*
>
> *John 5:44*

If you have to have other people validate you to feel good about yourself, you're a man pleaser. Worrying about other people's opinions is the fear of man. Fear is the opposite of faith. Fear is actually faith in a negative direction.

I was worried about what people thought of me. I was embarrassed and humiliated. That unbelief and fear negated my faith. Yes, I had faith. But I also had unbelief. I was still swayed by what people thought about me, and it canceled my faith.

"Let Her Go!"

God began to reveal this truth to me while I was reading a book about Smith Wigglesworth. He used to start each one of his meetings by standing up on the platform and boldly declaring, "Whoever gets up here first will be healed of whatever disease you've got." Then he would minister to them and see them healed. This would get everybody's attention, and he would teach on how it happened. Afterward he'd have a prayer line and pray for multitudes of people.

A couple of women in the front row knew his pattern, so they popped right up as soon as he made this invitation. Between them, they had an elderly friend who was so weak and frail that she hadn't even been able to sit up by herself, much less stand. There had to be one lady on each side of her to hold her up. The large tumor she had on her belly made her appear to be nine months pregnant. She was in very bad shape, so at Smith's declaration, the two ladies grabbed her and stuck her up on the platform.

There these two women were—one on either side holding up the woman who had this huge tumor. Wigglesworth looked at them and said, "Let her go."

At first, the ladies explained to him, "We can't let her go. She's too weak, and can't stand up on her own."

As Wigglesworth was known to do, he yelled at them, "I said let her go!" So they did. That woman fell flat on her face on top of that tumor, and let out a loud groan of pain.

The audience gasped, full of shock and unbelief, which was the same response I had received when I pulled that man out of his wheelchair. In this similar situation, I had responded with guilt, shame, and fear of what other people thought. I was thinking, *Lawsuit!* and all of these other terrible things. How did Smith Wigglesworth respond? He said, "Pick her up."

So they picked this woman up, and once they had her standing again between them, Smith said, "Let her go." It didn't faze him one bit. He wasn't moved off of his faith.

Less Unbelief

The two ladies answered him, "We will not let her go! We can't let her go. She'll fall."

He yelled at them again, saying, "Let her go!" So they let her go. A second time this lady fell on her face on top of that tumor. The people in the audience were shocked. Moans and groans of unbelief rippled throughout the entire audience. Wigglesworth wasn't phased; he said, "Pick her up." So they picked her up. Then he said, "Let her go."

These women protested, "We will not let her go!"

He yelled, "You let her go!"

A man in the audience stood up and said, "You beast! Leave that poor woman alone!"

Wigglesworth answered, "I know my business. You mind your own." Then he turned back to those ladies and roared, "LET HER GO!" They let her go. She started to fall, but then caught herself. That tumor fell right out of her dress onto the stage, and she walked off perfectly healed.

The Lord showed me that Smith Wigglesworth didn't have any more faith than I had. (Romans 12:3.) He didn't get any better results that first time he ministered to this woman than I got when I pulled that man out of his wheelchair. She fell flat on her face, just like he did. What was the difference? Smith didn't have any more faith, he just had less unbelief. He didn't care what people thought about him.

In fact, the book said that Smith was often criticized as being harsh and hard. Do you know what the word hard means in reference to our emotions? It means cold, insensitive, unfeeling, or unyielding to what other people think. The difference between Smith and me wasn't that he had more faith. He had less sensitivity to people's criticism. He was hardened toward what others thought. He wasn't responding to anybody or anything except what God had told him. I was still too dominated by people's opinions, by my physical realm, and what I could see, taste, hear, smell, and feel. So the difference wasn't that Smith had more faith; it was that he had less unbelief.

Decrease Your Unbelief

Most people don't understand this truth. When they pray for someone to be healed, but don't immediately see the manifestation, they often think, *I just don't have enough faith.* So they start trying to build and increase their faith. They have this misconception that they need to have a huge faith. However, this violates what Jesus taught in Matthew 17:20 when He said, "If your faith is the size of a tiny, little mustard seed, that's enough to remove a mountain into the sea." In other words, He was saying, "Guys, you don't need big faith. What you need is a pure faith that doesn't have anything contradicting, counteracting, or negating it. You need a faith that doesn't have anything pulling it in an opposite direction." Most people don't deal with unbelief in their life. Instead, they try to build faith.

Unbelief comes very similar to the way that faith does.

So then faith cometh by hearing, and hearing by the word of God.

Romans 10:17

In other words, faith comes when we focus our attention on God and His Word. Unbelief comes in a similar way, but from the opposite direction. Unbelief comes when we focus our attention on what people have to say. It comes when we listen to all the negative things the doctor has to say. If we consider, ponder, and think on all of those negatives, they'll negate our faith. So the key to the Christian life isn't learning how to develop a huge faith, it's learning how to decrease the amount of unbelief in our life. Very few Christians have this understanding.

Most Christians will spend an extra hour a day in the Word trying to build their faith. But then, during the day, they wash it down with two or three hours' worth of "As the Stomach Turns" on television and reading through all the bad news in the newspaper. They'll allow all this sewage from the world to flow through them—thoughts, attitudes, and concepts that are completely contrary to God's Word—and then they wonder why their faith isn't working.

You don't need a huge faith. You just need a pure faith that isn't counterbalanced by everything else.

How did Smith Wigglesworth get to where his faith wasn't polluted by unbelief? He resisted unbelief by refusing to focus on anything but God's Word.

One day Lester Sumrall[1] knocked on Smith Wigglesworth's door. He asked Smith if he could come in to visit. Smith told him he could come in, but the paper under his arm had to stay outside. Smith never read the newspaper and refused one to be brought into his house.

Some people say, "That's really narrow-minded." Well, it is. I agree that there are some good things in the newspaper. Over the years, I've used some newspaper articles to verify a point in my messages. I believe that over Smith's thirty-five year ministry he probably missed a dozen or so good things he could have used in his sermons. But it's certain he missed thousands of bad things that would have opened the door to unbelief. If you're going to go overboard, that's the side to do it on.

Abraham Considered Not

Consider how Abraham believed God.

Who against hope believed in hope, that he might become the father of many nations, according to that which was spoken, So shall thy seed be. And being not weak in faith, he considered not his own body now dead, when he was about an hundred years old, neither yet the deadness of Sara's womb: He staggered not at the promise of God through unbelief; but was strong in faith, giving glory to God; And being fully persuaded that, what he had promised, he was able also to perform.

Romans 4:18–21

This passage of scripture reveals that Abraham wasn't weak in faith because he *considered not* his own body now dead. He didn't have a big, huge faith, but he did have a faith that wasn't negated and counterbalanced by unbelief. Abraham simply didn't consider anything that was contrary to what God had said.

Speaking also of Abraham, Hebrews 11 says:

Truly, if they had been mindful of that country from whence they came out, they might have had opportunity to have returned.

Hebrews 11:15

If Abraham and Sarah's minds had been full of thoughts of the country they had left behind in obedience to God, they would have been tempted to return. In other words, your temptation is linked to what you think.

You need to understand this; it will change your life if you understand and apply it. You cannot be tempted with what you don't think. You have to think about something before you can be tempted with it. Therefore, you cannot be tempted with unbelief unless you think thoughts of unbelief. We need to quit listening to everyone else and all of their unbelief. We need to stop considering the negativism, cynicism, and anti-God/anti-Christ sentiment of this world. If we didn't listen to those thoughts, we wouldn't be tempted to disbelieve God.

Through many years of ministry, I've found that the hardest people to be healed out of all the professions are doctors, nurses, and those who have received medical training. Personally, I believe the reason is that they have been taught certain ways. It's not that everything medical professionals are taught is evil. It's just that it is presented to and hammered into them as fact.

Their instructors tell them facts like, "Here's what happens when a person gets a tumor; when it gets to this stage, then they will die." But they never finish by saying, "Unless they receive healing from God." They don't ever present the medical training in a spiritual context and show that God is capable of overcoming anything. So, over and over again medical students keep receiving the teaching of facts like, *When a tumor is at this stage, the person will die. They will have so many weeks to live, and that's it. It's incurable.* And by the time they finish school, it is engrained in their thoughts.

I've had some medical professionals come and try to receive their healing, and they just can't understand why it is so hard for them. It's because they have been taught so much unbelief, and it negates their little mustard seed of faith.

Chapter 14

A Pure, Strong Faith

In Matthew 17:20, Jesus was saying, "Guys, you don't have a faith problem. What you have is an unbelief problem." The parallel account in Mark 9 says that:

> *They brought him unto him: and when he saw him, straightway the spirit tare him; and he fell on the ground, and wallowed foaming.*
>
> *Mark 9:20*

Personally, I believe this is what caused their unbelief. If you've ever seen an epileptic seizure, you know that it can be a frightful experience, especially if the person starts biting or swallowing their tongue. It's terrible. I'm not trying to be cold-hearted or cruel, but I've seen it before. It can make the hair rise up on the back of your head.

These disciples had faith. They had seen other demons cast out and people healed, but this time, when they went to pray for this boy, there was a physical manifestation of these demons. The same thing happened to Jesus when He went to minister to this lad. The difference was Jesus had zero unbelief to counter His faith, so He was able to go ahead and effect a cure. These disciples, however, had responded in unbelief, which negated their faith. As a result, when they asked the Lord, "Why could we not cast him out? We know we were believing. We've seen it happen before, but how come it didn't work this time?" He told them, "It's because of your unbelief. Your unbelief negated, canceled out, and counterbalanced your faith."

Then in Matthew 17:21, Jesus continued by saying:

Howbeit this kind [of unbelief] goeth not out but by prayer and fasting.

Contrary to much popular teaching, and now even a few erroneous Bible versions, the true subject of verse 21 is the unbelief mentioned in verse 20, not the demon(s) in verse 19. Some people teach that certain demons are stronger than others, and that you must pray and fast in order to be able to cast them out. There are all kinds of variations on this, but it is not what Matthew 17:21 is saying. If you look carefully, you'll see that the subject of the previous sentence (v. 20) was *unbelief*, not *demons*. Unbelief was what stopped the disciples from casting out this demon and seeing the boy healed. And since the Lord said, "This kind only goes out through much prayer and fasting," apparently there are different kinds of unbelief.

Let me quickly mention that one of the same translations that substitutes "little faith" for "unbelief" in verse 20, totally leaves out verse 21. I'm not quick to criticize translations. I'm aware that many people don't like the *King James Version* that I use. However, any translation that omits verses is not what I consider good. You need a good translation of the Bible. Check yours out to see if Matthew 17:21 and Mark 16:17–20 are there.

Three Kinds of Unbelief

This is just "Andy-ology," but through my study of the Word and experience in ministry, it seems to me that there are three different kinds of unbelief.

First, there is unbelief that comes from *ignorance*. Sometimes people oppose what God says not because of anything specific, but because of a lack of knowledge. They just don't know any better. They don't know that God wants you well. They've never heard that truth before. It's ignorance, but nonetheless it's unbelief.

The way to overcome this first kind of unbelief—ignorance—is to tell people the truth. Show them the truth of God's Word. If they respect His Word, and are sensitive to His Spirit, they'll receive the knowledge they need to overcome this unbelief.

The second type of unbelief comes from *wrong doctrine*. Many people nowadays have been taught wrong. They've been told, "God doesn't do miracles today. Healing isn't for us today. These things passed away with the apostles." That's not true. It's not what the Word of God teaches. But nonetheless, it's what they have been taught.

This unbelief that comes from wrong teaching is harder to overcome than just ignorance. That's because you must first counter the wrong doctrine, and then teach them the truth. The antidote is exactly the same as for the first kind of unbelief. It just takes an extra step administering it—sitting down with them and countering their objections. The answer for both of these first two types of unbelief is to receive the truth of God's Word.

117

Then there's a third type of unbelief that I call *natural unbelief*. It's unbelief that comes from natural information that is contrary to God's Word. If you pray for someone to be healed and they fall over dead, your eyes, your ears, and all of your senses are going to tell you, "It didn't work." That's not necessarily because of ignorance or wrong doctrine. It's just that you've learned to trust what you see, taste, hear, smell, and feel. If you pray for your body to quit hurting, yet you can still feel pain, your body is going to be giving you thoughts of natural unbelief. It's not demonic or evil. Your five senses aren't of the devil. They have an important place and function in our everyday life.

Develop Your Sixth Sense

If you were going to drive me somewhere, I wouldn't want you to drive your car by faith. I'd want you to open up your eyes and see if there is another vehicle coming before proceeding through that intersection. That's not wrong or acting in unbelief. But if you know God has spoken something to you by the Word and/or by His Spirit, and your physical senses are telling you, "It's not going to work," then you have to be able to go beyond those five senses. When God wants you to do something contrary to what you can see, taste, hear, smell, and feel, then your five natural senses can give you thoughts of unbelief that can negate your faith.

This is what happened with the disciples in Matthew 17. They saw a physical manifestation of this demon that was contrary to what they were praying and believing for, and it caused them to fear. Their five senses ministered thoughts of unbelief that countered their faith.

It was miraculous how I saw that first man raised from the dead. I didn't know what was wrong when I walked into the room. I was standing right in front of the man before I realized he was dead. I heard his wife crying, "Oh, God. Bring Everett back from the dead." When she said that, it was the first time I had even had a thought that the guy was dead. When I heard her prayer, I just looked at the man and commanded, "Everett, in the name of Jesus, come back into your body." Then he just sat up. It was that simple.

It would have been much more difficult if I would have had thirty minutes to think about him being dead. If somebody would have told me what I was going over there to pray for, my mind would probably have come up with enough thoughts of unbelief to negate and counterbalance my faith. Personally, I believe that one of the reasons I saw this man raised from the dead was because I just didn't have time to think about anything else.

These disciples had already seen demons cast out and people healed. Apparently, they hadn't faced a physical manifestation like this before. Therefore, they hadn't had the same temptation to unbelief. But in this instance, there was a physical manifestation contrary to what they'd prayed for, and it caused them thoughts of unbelief. Understanding this, Jesus told them, "The only way you can get rid of this natural kind of unbelief is through fasting and prayer. It's not just a matter of studying the Word more.

You need to get into the presence of God and renew yourself to such a degree that you develop your sixth sense, which is faith."

Fasting and Prayer

This is important. You have five senses—what you can see, taste, hear, smell, and feel. If one of those senses were to be damaged, let's say you went blind, you could still get around. What you'd have to do is depend more upon your other remaining senses, like hearing and feeling. You would have to listen to what's happening around you, and use a cane to touch and feel the variances in the ground ahead as you walk along. You could still get around and walk places, but you'd have to rely more on your other senses.

Some blind people memorize what their apartment is like, and where everything is. They can walk in the dark because they aren't using their eyes. They're using their ears and touch primarily. So you can compensate for losing one of your senses by depending on the others more.

What happens when God reveals to you through His Word that it is His will to heal you, but all five of your senses are telling you, "It didn't work. I still feel pain. I still look sick. I still have this and that, and I can taste something in my mouth that shows me I haven't been healed yet"? If all five of your senses are telling you it didn't work, you need to develop a sixth sense that will tell you it did work. That sixth sense is *faith*.

You can get to where you actually believe that you have faith, and that faith becomes as real to you as what you can see, taste, hear, smell, and feel. You do that by spending time in the spiritual realm. That's what prayer and fasting are all about.

Fasting doesn't change God. It doesn't make Him move. Fasting and prayer don't make demons leave. There is no demon that you will ever encounter that will require fasting and prayer added to what Jesus has already done to cast them out. If you encounter a demon and it doesn't respond to the name of Jesus and faith in His name, then your prayer and fasting isn't going to get them out either. Speaking the Word of God and the name of Jesus in faith will deal with any demon. So, your fasting and prayer doesn't move God. Neither does it move the devil. Fasting and prayer moves you. It affects you.

Your appetite is one of the strongest desires your flesh has. When you deny your flesh by fasting, it's going to rise up and rebel because it wants to be fed. Your flesh wants to be indulged and taken care of. If you tell your flesh, "No! Man doesn't eat by bread alone, but by every word that proceeds from the mouth of God" (Matthew 4:4; Luke 4:4), I can guarantee you that your flesh is going to rebel. Although you'll think you are dying by noon the first day, it's not true. If you persevere, after awhile your body and your senses will begin to learn. They'll say, "Hey, I didn't die at noon." As a matter of fact, after fasting about three days, you'll get to where you aren't hungry any more.

You may not have experienced this yet, but it's true. You can literally bring your five senses under control, and they'll begin to recognize that, "Hey, I'm not going to starve. Okay, this faith stuff is real." You really can be sustained by God, and not by food alone. You can teach your flesh that.

Then when you say to your body, "You're healed in Jesus' name," your flesh may answer, "I still hurt," but that sixth sense says "I'm healed and I believe it. So okay, I've experienced this before." But if you haven't spent time fasting, praying, and being in the presence of God, your body will say, "No, I still hurt." You'll say, "Body, you get in line," but your flesh will answer, "Who are you to tell me what to do? I tell you when to eat, what to eat, and how much to eat." It's just like a spoiled brat. But you can train your senses to discern both good (God and His Word) and evil (what contradicts them).

> *Strong meat belongeth to them that are of full age, even those who by reason of use have their senses exercised to discern both good and evil.*
>
> *Hebrews 5:14*

You can get to the place where someone like Smith Wigglesworth lived, listening to what faith has to say more than what natural things like your mind, emotions, senses, and circumstances have to say. When you do that, you're decreasing in unbelief.

The Measure of Faith

According to Romans 4, it's more biblically accurate to say that, depending on the level of unbelief, you either have a weak faith or a strong faith.

> *And being not weak in faith, he considered not his own body now dead, when he was about an hundred years old, neither yet*

the deadness of Sara's womb: He staggered not at the promise
of God through unbelief; but was strong in faith, giving glory
to God; And being fully persuaded that, what he had promised,
he was able also to perform.

Romans 4:19–21

What you're doing is describing how much unbelief you have mixed with your faith. If you have a lot of unbelief, then you're weak in faith. If you have little unbelief, then you're strong in faith. That's an appropriate description. Whereas, little faith and big faith isn't really appropriate. The truth is every one of us has been given the faith of the Son of God.

God hath dealt to every man the measure of faith.

Romans 12:3

Knowing that a man is not justified by the works of the law,
but by the faith of Jesus Christ, even we have believed in Jesus
Christ, that we might be justified by the faith of Christ, and
not by the works of the law: for by the works of the law shall
no flesh be justified…I am crucified with Christ: nevertheless
I live; yet not I, but Christ liveth in me: and the life which I
now live in the flesh I live by the faith of the Son of God, who
loved me, and gave himself for me.

Galatians 2:16,20

For further study of this important foundational truth, I encourage you to check out my teaching entitled, *"The Faith of God."* It's available both as a single message and as the third part of *Spirit, Soul & Body.*

123

Every born-again Christian has the exact same amount and quality of faith that Jesus had. You don't have a faith problem. What you have is an unbelief problem. Instead of trying to build bigger and bigger faith, we need to stop feeding unbelief. We need to turn off the sources of unbelief in our life and starve our unbelief. We need to get to where we spend so much time in the spiritual world thinking on God and the truths of His Word that we don't even have the same thoughts of unbelief.

Let's be like Abraham, who didn't even consider the fact that he was a hundred years old and his wife was ninety. He just thought about what God had promised him, which was that they were going to have a child. Romans 4:19 says that Abraham didn't even consider his own body now dead, neither yet the deadness of Sarah's womb. This enabled him not to stagger in unbelief at the promise of God.

The Key to Victory

When it comes to ministering healing, it's not usually that people don't have faith. Some don't, but most do. However, they also have unbelief. Therefore, their faith is weak. It's canceled out, negated, and counterbalanced by unbelief. The reason is that they haven't been spending time in the presence of God. They are so accustomed to the world, they're thinking thoughts of unbelief. They're thinking, "It's flu season. Everyone else has it," or "My father died from this same thing that's fighting me." They consider, ponder, and think about all these natural things, and that unbelief negates their faith.

So the key to victory in the Christian life isn't necessarily having huge faith, it's having a simple, pure, childlike faith—faith the size of a mustard seed—that isn't canceled out by unbelief. You need to unhook from the unbelief that is pulling you in the opposite direction, and let your little mustard seed amount of faith pull you to victory.

Some folks think that the only reason people aren't healed is because they don't have any faith. That offends other people who'll argue, "No, this person loved God. They were a great person of faith." They'll summarily dismiss your criticism saying, "It must not be God's will to heal." However, you now know that this isn't all there is to it. You can have faith, love God, and be a great person, yet have unbelief that pulls you in the other direction.

Starve your unbelief. Get to where you are so single-minded about the Lord and His Word that your little mustard seed amount of faith will be enough to accomplish anything you need. Like a leech or a fungus, unbelief has to be fed and nourished. Separate yourself even for a week. Fasting, praying, and focusing your attention on the Lord can do great damage to your unbelief. It doesn't cause God to give you more power. It just causes the faith you have to work so much better because you are diminishing the unbelief that's pulling in the opposite direction. That's good news!

Once you believe the truth that God wants you well, then all you have to do is starve the unbelief until your faith starts producing the results you desire.

Chapter 15

Governed by Law

So far we have learned that healing is part of Christ's atonement, which means it's not optional. It's already been provided for. The Lord would no more withhold healing from us than He would withhold forgiveness of sin. Our sins have been forgiven and our bodies have been healed by the one atonement of our Lord Jesus Christ.

We need to get this attitude that our healing has already been accomplished. If we were to fight for it the same as we fight to resist sin, then we would see a marked difference in the number of people who receive healing. However, many folks are passive when it comes to healing. They pray a prayer like, "Lord, heal me, if it be Your will." That is absolutely inaccurate because the Word says:

> *Beloved, I wish above all things that thou mayest prosper and be in health, even as thy soul prospereth.*
>
> *3 John 2*

The word "wish" here means that it is His will. God's will is for us to be well. Once we see His will revealed plainly like this in His Word, there's no reason for us to pray any longer "If it be Your will." It's a matter of appropriating healing—reaching out in faith, taking, and receiving. It's standing in faith for the full manifestation. We have to be aggressive and fight to receive what God has given. We must not allow the world, the flesh, or the devil to deny us what Jesus has already provided.

Life and Peace

Sickness is never a blessing. God's Word is very clear. We saw earlier that Deuteronomy 28:1–14 lists what God considers a blessing and that verses 16–68 reveals what He considers a curse. Sickness and disease are always a curse. For religion to come along and teach that sickness is actually a blessing from God is a perversion of what His Word says.

Yes, the Lord did smite some people with sickness in the Old Testament. However, there's a huge difference between the Old Covenant and the New. God doesn't smite people like that in the New Covenant. But remember, even under the law, sickness was always a curse—never a blessing. And Christ has redeemed us from the curse of the law (Galatians 3:12–13), which includes everything listed in Deuteronomy 28:16–68.

The reason why most people aren't healed is unbelief in one form or another. Unbelief is a counterbalancing, opposing force to faith. Most people try to build and increase faith, but do nothing about the amount of their unbelief. They simply don't understand that faith and unbelief are opposing forces. Jesus said in Matthew 17:20 that a mustard seed amount of faith is all we need to do anything, even see a mountain cast into the sea.

We don't have a faith problem. What we really have is an unbelief problem. We expose ourselves to all kinds of thoughts, attitudes, feelings, and emotions that war against our faith. To have a strong faith, we need to decrease the amount of unbelief in our life by taking our focus away from the world and away from anything that contradicts God's Word, especially in the area of healing. We need to quit listening to all the negative reports and focus on the Word of God. If all our thoughts are spiritually minded, then all we'll get is life and peace. (Romans 8:6.)

Constant and Universal

The kingdom of God—including faith—operates by law. Understanding this truth is essential to walking in divine health.

I go more in-depth on this truth and how it applies specifically to healing in such teachings as *How to Receive a Miracle* and *You've Already Got It!* I encourage you to get them.

A law is consistent and universal. It's always the same, and never fluctuates, anywhere you go. Anything that doesn't fit that criteria isn't a law, but a phenomenon. Take, for instance, gravity. Gravity is a law. We call it the law of gravity. It's always constant. It always works. It's always the same no matter where you go. If gravity only worked in the United States, but over in Europe, Africa, or Asia there was weightlessness, then it would be a phenomenon, not a law. If gravity only manifested sometimes, and other times there was weightlessness, it would be a phenomenon. But when something is consistent and universal, then that means it is a law.

God created this world and the laws that govern it. In addition to gravity, there are laws concerning such things as electricity and inertia. The law of inertia tells us that once an object is in motion, it tends to stay in motion. Once inertia has built up, it takes time and effort to overcome. That's why you have to apply the brakes in order to stop a moving car. How long it takes to stop depends on how fast you're going and the size and mass of the vehicle. This is the law of inertia. It also works when you're sitting still. Inertia works against you, and it takes time to accelerate and get a car moving from a stopped position. But once it's rolling you can coast. These are just a few examples of the different laws in effect.

God created these laws—both natural and spiritual—and He doesn't violate them. This truth directly applies to healing.

Intended for Our Good

I constantly talk with people who simply don't understand that the spiritual realm is governed by laws. They don't look at the kingdom of God as being governed by laws. They honestly think that the Lord just does anything He wants.

Many people take up an offense against God when someone in their family dies. They say, "Why didn't God heal this person? If He wanted to, He could have." They fail to understand that there are laws that govern His kingdom.

In the physical realm, the law of gravity applies even to the person who walks off the edge of a tall building. God doesn't want that person to die. He actually created gravity to be a positive force in our life. Right now, I'm sitting in a chair. I don't have to strap myself in or hold myself down. I don't have to be bolted to the floor because gravity is working. However, that same law that's meant for our good will kill us if we walk off a ten-story building. God didn't create gravity to harm us. He made it to help us function here on planet earth. The whole world functions that way, and it's good. But if someone violates the laws God created—like stepping off a tall building—the same force that God intended for our good will kill us.

Some folks argue that if the Lord wanted to, He could just stop that. However, God doesn't just change the laws. That's not His nature. When He created these laws as part of the original creation, He said, "It is very good." (Genesis 1:31.) There's nothing wrong with gravity. The problem isn't with the law. It's with the people who violate these laws. If God suspended the law of gravity to save one life, think of the untold millions of other lives that would be lost because of that suspension. People depending on gravity to hold their car to the road while driving would suddenly careen out of control into other cars and buildings. Millions of people would die just so He could save the life of one person falling off of a building. It doesn't work that way.

Laws are constant. They don't fluctuate. God doesn't violate natural laws. He doesn't violate spiritual laws either. There are spiritual laws, and they are intended for our good. The Lord has designed things so that it's not just on His whim that people are

131

healed. There are laws that govern faith and healing. There are reasons why things happen the way that they do. Our ignorance of these laws, and of the truth that there are these laws, is a huge hindrance to receiving healing. Ignorance of what these individual laws are will hinder people from receiving healing, even those who understand that the kingdom of God is operated and governed by laws.

Electricity

Electricity has been around since God created the earth. There's a magnetic field in the earth and electricity in the air. You can see that especially in cold, dry climates when you walk on a carpet and then touch a doorknob. The static electricity will shock you. These kinds of things have happened since the first day that God created the earth. I heard someone say that there's enough energy in a typical thunderstorm to power the city of New York for one whole year.

God didn't just choose to give electricity to man a few hundred years ago. No, electricity has been here from the beginning. It was man's ignorance of electricity that kept him from being able to use it the way we do today. God didn't hold him back. If man would have understood the laws that govern electricity, and learned how to cooperate with them, we could have enjoyed the benefits of electricity thousands of years ago. Jesus and His disciples could have used the air conditioners, washing machines, and dishwashers we use today. The potential has always been there. It was just our ignorance that kept us from it.

Likewise, there are things that men are dreaming about inventing right now. Many of these ideas sound far-fetched to us today, but they're possible. God isn't holding us back. It's our own ignorance of the laws. We're still in the process of discovering, and many radical changes are yet to come.

Consider the huge changes in telecommunications that have taken place in just the past few years alone. Today, nearly everyone has a cell phone. There's no reason why people couldn't have been talking on cell phones 2,000 years ago. Both the materials to make the cell phones, and the natural laws that govern how they work, have been here on the earth from the beginning of time. God wasn't holding us back. We were ignorant of the laws. The ability was there, but we had to understand how to operate it.

There is a natural fear of things we don't understand. You may understand how to flip a switch and make a light turn on, but you don't know all the laws governing electricity's use. Electricity can kill, and people who don't understand it are fearful of it.

Personally, I don't fully understand electricity. When I do electrical work, I go to the breaker box and shut off all the breakers in the whole house. Now, I know you don't have to do that, but one time when I just shut off one breaker, there happened to be an adjacent breaker box that was grounded to the one I was working on, and the electricity knocked me flat on my back!

Another time, I was helping do a total remodel on someone's bathroom. I was working on replacing all the fixtures, and was

133

about to go turn off all of the breakers in the whole house. A man came in and said, "You don't even have to turn off the breakers at all." He then proceeded to work with the live wires. We had just pulled out the sink, and there was water on the floor. He just stood there in the water working with the wires, and he never got shocked. Some people think, *You can't do that!* You can if you know what you are doing. Since I don't know enough about electricity and how it works to do something like that, I have a natural fear and inability that someone who understands and operates in that knowledge doesn't have.

The Law of Faith

It's the same way in the spiritual world. There are reasons why some people are able to walk in the power of God, and others aren't. Basically, God's Word is His manual that tells us what these laws are and how His kingdom operates.

> *Where is boasting then? It is excluded. By what law? of works? Nay: but by the law of faith.*
>
> *Romans 3:27*

Although this verse in context is actually talking about the tension between grace and faith, we can also see an important principle here in the final phrase. Notice the terminology: "the law of faith."

Faith is governed by law. So when a person has need of healing, it's not a matter of just petitioning God, and then if He wants them healed they'll be healed. No, that's not it. There are laws that govern how healing works. It's primarily our ignorance of God's laws and how His kingdom works that keeps His power from operating. Most people simply don't see that the kingdom of God is established on laws, and laws are consistent. God doesn't change. Neither does He violate His own laws just because people don't understand this.

Many people get angry at God when somebody dies or a healing doesn't manifest. They think, *If He wanted to, He could have healed me.* God certainly has the power, but that power doesn't flow independent of His laws. There are spiritual laws that govern how faith works and how the power of God flows. If we don't know that, then we stop the power of God and do without because of our ignorance.

Some people take offense when they first hear these truths. They say, "You're criticizing me!" Well, I am, but in the same way that I would criticize Leonardo da Vinci. In his day, da Vinci was considered a genius. He actually invented many things hundreds of years before we had the ability to make them. For instance, people have applied modern technology that Leonardo didn't have, like electric motors and lighter materials, and built a working helicopter based on his designs. Although he lived in the 1400s, this man was way ahead of his time.

Many of da Vinci's concepts and plans didn't work back then because he didn't have access to what we know and have today. He didn't use electricity. He didn't have the benefit of electrical motors, and the like. Yet, this man was a genius. When I point out that he was ignorant of the laws governing electricity, I'm not saying he was stupid. I'm just stating that he lacked knowledge in certain areas. He didn't understand some of the things that we understand and take for granted today.

Still Growing

I am not criticizing or trying to put down anyone when I say that a lot of people are ignorant of the laws of God. I'm simply pointing out the truth that there are many things available to us from God that we don't receive because we don't understand and cooperate with the laws of His kingdom.

Through studying the Word, I've discovered a number of these laws that govern how the kingdom of God works. However, I am convinced that there is much more that I still don't understand. That's the reason why things don't work any better for me than they do. Although I don't know everything, I could probably tell you at least a hundred different laws and principles I've found concerning healing. Still, there are other laws that I don't yet understand, which is why while I don't see every single person healed, I have seen lots of people healed. I am growing and working on this.

Chapter 16

The Spiritual World

The account of the woman with the issue of blood vividly illustrates several of these spiritual laws concerning healing. This isn't an all-inclusive list, but it's a great place to start.

> *And a certain woman, which had an issue of blood twelve years, And had suffered many things of many physicians, and had spent all that she had, and was nothing bettered, but rather grew worse, When she had heard of Jesus, came in the press behind, and touched his garment. For she said, If I may touch but his clothes, I shall be whole. And straightway the fountain of her blood was dried up; and she felt in her body that she was healed of that plague. And Jesus, immediately knowing in himself that virtue had gone out of him, turned him about in the press, and said, Who touched my clothes? And his disciples said unto him, Thou seest the multitude thronging thee, and sayest thou, Who touched me? And he looked round about to see her that had done this thing. But the woman fearing and trembling, knowing what was done in her, came and fell down before him, and told him all the truth. And he said unto her, Daughter, thy faith hath made thee whole; go in peace, and be whole of thy plague.*
>
> *Mark 5:25–34*

This passage shows us how the kingdom of God operates by law. When that woman came and touched the hem of Jesus' garment, He felt virtue—power—go out of Him. So He asked, "Who touched My clothes?" Immediately, His disciples began to say, "You see the crowd of people pressing in to touch You." In other words, this multitude of people weren't just casually bumping up against Jesus. They were trying to touch Him because they recognized the power and virtue that was in Him. Therefore, many people were touching Him. The disciples said, "Why are You asking who touched You? Everybody is touching You." But Jesus could tell a difference.

"Who Touched Me?"

Some people think that asking this question, "Who touched Me?" was actually deceptive on God's part. They assume that since Jesus was God that He certainly knew all things, including who had touched Him. They argue that He was just saying this as a way to try to get this woman to come forward voluntarily. That's not true.

Many people don't understand this truth that Jesus was both fully God and fully man. He was 100 percent God in His spirit, but His physical body was human—sinless human, but human nonetheless. Our Lord took upon Himself a human body, and Luke 2:52 reveals that:

Jesus increased in wisdom and stature, and in favour with God and man.

Jesus had to grow up and learn things. In His spirit, as God, He knew all things. But since He was living in a physical body, His physical body had to learn. He didn't come out of the womb speaking Hebrew, understanding math, and practicing carpentry. Jesus had to learn how to eat, walk, and talk just the same as other children do. He was sinless, but He was human, and He had to grow.

The physical realm of Jesus had limitations. His physical body could only be in one place at one time, and it grew tired.

> *Hast thou not known? hast thou not heard, that the everlasting God, the LORD, the Creator of the ends of the earth, fainteth not, neither is weary? there is no searching of his understanding.*

> *Isaiah 40:28*

Since Jesus grew tired at times, does that mean He wasn't God? No, He was God in His spirit, but His physical body had limitations. Therefore, when Jesus asked, "Who touched Me?" in His physical being, He didn't know who had touched Him.

Already Approved

Many people think that God just sovereignly looks over things. When someone gets healed, it's because they gave their request to God and He granted it. They visualize God in heaven sitting behind a desk piled high with prayers. Their petition goes by and He either stamps "Approved" or "Disapproved" on it. So if someone gets healed it's because God had mercy on them and healed them. If they don't, it's because He chose not to heal them for whatever reason. This attitude is expressed again and again as people say, "Why didn't God heal so and so? I prayed for them. He could have done it." They think that it's up to God to approve or disapprove of our healing. The truth is, through the stripes on Jesus' back, God has already approved all our healing.

> *Who his own self bare our sins in his own body on the tree,*
> *that we, being dead to sins, should live unto righteousness: by*
> *whose stripes ye were [past tense] healed.*
>
> *1 Peter 2:24*

Through Christ's death, burial, and resurrection, He has already paid for every person's healing. He's already stamped "Approved". It's not now up to God; there are laws through which our faith has to function. The healing He's already provided for us won't flow until we learn these laws and begin to put them into practice.

Flip the Switch

The spiritual world operates on spiritual laws the same way the natural world operates on natural laws.

Electricity is generated by the power company. It's delivered to where you work and live by power lines. However, if you want your lights on, you don't call the electric company and ask, "Could you please turn my lights on? Andrew Wommack is coming over and we're having a meeting here tonight." It doesn't matter what your need or desire is because the electric company has already done their part. They have supplied you with the power, but it's at your command. The power company isn't going to send someone out to flip the switch on your wall to turn the light on. That's not their job. They generate the power and supply it to you. But you are the one who has to turn it on.

It's the same way in the spiritual world. God has already provided His healing power for everyone. Jesus has already healed you. By His stripes, you were already healed. (1 Peter 2:24.) If you are just praying and waiting on God to do something, then you are violating the laws that govern faith. You aren't cooperating with the kingdom. God has already provided healing. If you are a born-again Christian, the same virtue that raised Jesus Christ from the dead already dwells on the inside of you. You don't have a problem with God generating the power and making it available to you in your born-again spirit. The problem is that you haven't learned how to activate and release it into manifestation. You haven't yet learned how to flip the switch and turn it on. You aren't cooperating with God by faith.

You could call the power company and wait all day for them to send someone to your house to flip the light switch, but they aren't going to do it. You could then say, "Well, the electricity doesn't work." No, it works just fine. You just don't know how to turn it on.

The Power Will Flow

Healing works. Jesus has already healed every person. He's already released the healing power. If someone isn't healed, it's not because Jesus hasn't given; it's because that person hasn't taken. He or she doesn't know how to turn on the power of God.

The woman with the issue of blood tapped into the power of God. She touched the hem of Jesus' garment, and virtue flowed—without the Lord looking at her and sizing her up to decide whether she was serious enough or not, whether she was holy enough or not, or any of the other criteria that religion claims about God. Jesus didn't do any of those things. Similar to electricity, the power just flowed.

If someone picked up a live wire that didn't have any insulation on it, the power would automatically flow through and shock them. It's not that the electric company shocked them personally to teach them a lesson. They were shocked because of the laws that govern electricity. If you touch a live wire, and you're grounded, then you're going to get shocked.

It's the same way with healing. You don't ever have to petition God. You don't have to beg, plead, and do all the things we've been taught that we have to do. All you must do is believe and reach out in faith to receive. If you are grounded in faith, the power will flow.

The woman with the issue of blood proved this. She put into motion the laws that govern faith, and the power of God flowed. Jesus didn't even know who had touched Him. Now, He did recognize the release of power. When He turned around and the woman wasn't forthcoming right away, I believe He drew on the gifts of the Holy Spirit and knew exactly who had touched Him. Then He was able to point this woman out (Mark 5:32) but it's significant to note here that Jesus didn't know who touched Him until after the power of God flowed. It wasn't God on a personal basis saying, "Yes, I will heal you," and stamping "Approved" on her prayer. No, the healing power is already generated and available. All you have to do is reach out and touch it in faith, and the power of God will flow.

Ignorance Is Deadly

This truth blesses and excites me. It answers a lot of questions for me. It tells me why certain good people who desired to be healed, were earnest in praying for it, died. God didn't reject them and their petition. The Lord didn't choose not to heal them. He has set up His kingdom to operate on laws. God wanted them healed and well, but they didn't cooperate.

To illustrate this concept, an inventor might have had some good ideas that he earnestly tried to invent and make work. He could come close, but there are laws. God couldn't say, "Oh well, you've come close. I'll just let this helicopter work even though you don't have the right materials. Even though you don't have a real power source, or even an electrical motor, you've been so sincere. Therefore, I'm going to let it work for you." No, there are natural laws that must be cooperated with. The inventor can be close, but close isn't close enough.

In the spiritual world, there are good people who petition God, but they just don't understand and cooperate with how the kingdom works. It's not God who rejected them, it's just that the kingdom operates by laws. If you violate those laws, they will kill you. Ignorance is deadly. In the natural realm, we say, "Ignorance is bliss. What you don't know won't hurt you."

143

That's not true, especially in the spiritual realm. What you don't know can kill you. (Hosea 4:6.) We need to understand how the kingdom of God works.

Faith Comes by Hearing

Let's take a closer look at this woman with the issue of blood. She understood and cooperated with several kingdom laws. First of all, she had to hear of Jesus.

> *A certain woman, which had an issue of blood twelve years, And had suffered many things of many physicians, and had spent all that she had, and was nothing bettered, but rather grew worse, When she had heard of Jesus, came in the press behind, and touched his garment.*
>
> *Mark 5:25–27*

Somebody told her about Jesus and the miracles He was performing. This basic law of faith is stated clearly in Romans:

> *So then faith cometh by hearing, and hearing by the word of God.*
>
> *Romans 10:17*

You have to hear about God. You must have information fed to you. God's Word feeds us information that is contrary to nearly all of the information that you'll get in the natural world. You won't have faith by listening to the (bad) news at night. You aren't going to get faith by watching soap operas on television, X-rated movies, and the like. Those things produce contrary information. If we want faith, we need to be in the Word of God.

She heard of God. She didn't necessarily hear about Jesus through reading the scriptures; but now we have the New Testament scriptures that include the ministry of Jesus, the ministry of His apostles, and revelation knowledge. If you are going to learn about Jesus today, you need to hear God's Word. You must get into and meditate on the Word of God.

This woman had heard about Jesus. She meditated, considered, and thought on what she had heard. She could have rejected it, but she received. Faith comes by hearing, and hearing by the Word of God.

Plug In to the Power Source

If you want to receive healing, you need to get into the Word of God. Psalm 107:20 says:

He sent his word, and healed them, and delivered them from their destructions.

God's Word will heal and deliver you. If you find it, it's life and health to all your flesh.

My son, attend to my words; incline thine ear unto my sayings. Let them not depart from thine eyes; keep them in the midst of thine heart. For they are life unto those that find them, and health to all their flesh.

Proverbs 4:20–22

This is one of God's laws that many people violate. They want to receive from the Lord, but they don't spend any time

145

in His Word. They may say, "Well, I believe that the Bible says somewhere that by His stripes we're healed, but I'm not sure if that's an exact quote or not." If that's how you are, you aren't going to get healed through the Word of God. Somebody else might minister to you, and you could get healed off their faith, but you aren't going to get healed being that vague. You need to know what the Word of God says. You need to be able to find the scriptures.

My teachings entitled *A Sure Foundation* and *Effortless Change* speak about the importance of God's Word, and how it works in our life.

If the Word of God isn't living on the inside of you, then you're violating one of the most foundational laws. That's like having a cord that isn't plugged in to any electrical outlet, yet wondering why your appliance isn't working. It's because you aren't plugged in to the power source. You need to plug in to the Word of God!

Chapter 17

Words Are Powerful

When the woman with the issue of blood had heard of Jesus, she…

Came in the press behind, and touched his garment. For she said, If I may touch but his clothes, I shall be whole.

Mark 5:27,28

Here she cooperated with another law: She spoke her faith. God's Word plainly and repeatedly reveals this truth in many different places, including Proverbs 18:

A man's belly shall be satisfied with the fruit of his mouth; and with the increase of his lips shall he be filled. Death and life are in the power of the tongue: and they that love it shall eat the fruit thereof.

Proverbs 18:20,21

Someone might cite Matthew's account of this same instance of the woman speaking her faith, where it says:

For she said within herself, If I may but touch his garment, I shall be whole.

Matthew 9:21

According to Matthew, she said this within herself, but according to Mark, she spoke with her mouth. Which is it? I believe it's both. Before we speak things out of our mouth, we say them within. The scriptures don't contradict each other. She did both, and this is one of the laws that govern faith.

Our words are powerful. With our words, we can release life, and with our words, we can release death. We need to recognize that there is power in our words—not only positive power, but also negative power.

Release Your Faith

If you are whining, griping, and complaining, you are releasing the negative force of unbelief. That unbelief will cancel out, counterbalance, and negate your faith. Many people pray and ask God to heal them. Then someone comes up to them and asks, "How are you?" They answer, "Oh, I'm dying. The doctor told me this and that, and everything in me hurts." They start speaking negative words—contrary to God's Word—with their mouth, and they're violating the laws governing faith.

That's like short circuiting an electrical current. The power may be there, but because you constantly short circuit it, it's not producing the desired results.

You must recognize that the words you speak are powerful. God created the heavens and the earth by words. He spoke the world into existence. He said, "Let there be light" (Genesis 1:3), and "Let the earth bring forth…fruit" (v. 11). The physical world, even your own physical body responds to words. Your words are important.

Many people think, *It doesn't matter what I say*, but God's Word reveals that it does matter what you say. What you say affects what you believe. It will affect your body, the devil, and even God. God uses your words. This is one of the most important ways that you release your faith.

Speak God's Word

In more than forty years of ministry, I've prayed for thousands of people. Over the years, I've learned that when I am praying for someone it's very important that I speak faith-filled words. I don't ever speak forth my doubts. There have been times when people have come to me in such bad shape that it caused fear and doubt to rise up inside me, but I never speak it. I only speak my faith. I've seen people healed in spite of my unbelief because I never spoke it.

Matthew 6:31 says:

Therefore take no thought, saying....

You can't keep a thought from coming, but you can keep from taking that thought as your own. "Take no thought, saying." You haven't really taken a thought until you begin to speak it forth. What you say is extremely important.

When this woman with the issue of blood said, "If I could but touch His clothes, I shall be made whole," she put a law of

God into motion. We just saw that there is death and life in the power of the tongue. She spoke something positive, and then, when she acted on it, the power was released.

If you are fighting some type of a sickness, you need to start speaking faith-filled words. You need to want the results of the words that you're saying. Don't just speak what the doctor has said, or how you feel. Speak what the Word of God says about you, and speak it in faith. At first you may not totally believe it, but faith comes by hearing— and hearing, and hearing—the Word of God. Speaking God's Word, and continuing to speak it, will help you to believe it.

Spiritual Power

Another passage of scripture that shows us the importance of our words is:

> *Verily I say unto you, That whosoever shall say unto this mountain, Be thou removed, and be thou cast into the sea; and shall not doubt in his heart, but shall believe that those things which he saith shall come to pass; he shall have whatsoever he saith.*
>
> *Mark 11:23*

Your words are emphasized three different times in this one verse. You must speak out your faith, not unbelief. When you speak your faith, spiritual power is released. It allows God to flow.

Most doctors have adopted this philosophy that they never want to get your hopes up. They always try to give you the worst-case scenario, thinking that's the good and wise thing to do. I'm aware that doctors do this for liability reasons, but you need to be getting people's hopes up and speaking positive words. You don't need to be speaking the negative things. When you're around somebody in a hospital room, don't talk to them about dying. Talk to them about living. Release life with your words. Speak the Word of God. His Word will become life and health to all their flesh. (Proverbs 4:22.)

Speak to Your Mountain

Again, Jesus said in Mark 11:23,

Whosoever shall say unto this mountain, Be thou removed.

The mountain mentioned here is referring to your problem. If you're sick and have a disease, speak to that disease. Say, "Cancer, you are dead. I command you out of my body in the name of Jesus. Cancer, you are leaving my body now." The Bible says to speak to your problem, yet most people speak to God about their problem. This is simple, but it's profound, and it has revolutionized my life.

When it comes to healing, you need to learn to operate in this principle. If you have a pain in your foot, say, "Pain in my foot, in Jesus' name I command you to leave." Don't say, "God, please take away the pain in my foot." That's not what He's instructed us to do. He told us to speak to our problem, not to speak to Him about our problem. Most people aren't cooperating with this truth. They are violating this law, and because of it the power of God doesn't flow. We need to do what the Lord has told us to do.

I remember ministering this truth to a woman with severe health problems in Charlotte, North Carolina. She was diagnosed in 1994 with all kinds of sickness and disease. She was in constant, excruciating pain, and suffered greatly. The doctors told her in 1997 that it was impossible for her to live much longer, and that she would die within a month. When I prayed for her, it was 2001. She had already gone four years beyond when they said she would die. However, she had a multitude of different things wrong with her, and lived in terrible pain.

I talked with her and explained some truths from the Word concerning healing. Then I prayed with her, and spoke to the pain. She had pain all throughout her body. So I commanded pain to leave. I didn't request it. I took my God-given authority as a believer and commanded pain to leave.

Take Authority and Command

This brings us to yet another important kingdom law. Since God has already done His part through Christ's atonement, *we need to take our authority as a believer and command the power of God to flow.* (Isaiah 45:11.) Instead of us asking with a question mark at the end of our sentence, wondering what God is going to do, we need to believe and act on the truth that the Lord has already done it. By His stripes, you were (past tense) healed (1 Peter 2:24).

So I spoke to that woman's body, I spoke to the pain, and I commanded it to leave. Instantly, she was free of pain for the first time in seven years. She started praising God, but then stopped and said, "I still have a burning in my back right along my waist. How come this burning didn't leave?"

I responded, "Well, I didn't speak to burning. You didn't tell me about a burning, so I didn't speak to that." So I prayed again, and this time I said, "Burning, in the name of Jesus, I command you to leave." And it left.

This woman was just beside herself, walking around and praising God. I spent almost a half an hour telling her how to keep her healing because Satan will come and try to steal the Word away. (Mark 4:15.) I told her what to do if she ever had another pain, burning, or anything like that.

How the Kingdom Works

Sure enough, before she got ready to leave, she looked at me and said, "The burning has come back."

I said, "Well, I've already told you how to do it. I'm going to join hands with you and agree, but you do the praying. You take charge of this thing."

So this woman prayed a pretty good prayer, saying, "Father, I thank You that it is Your will to heal me." Thirty minutes before she had believed that God was the One who had given her this sickness. But she had received God's Word when I countered that unbelief. She prayed, "Father, I believe that by Your stripes I

153

was healed. I claim my healing in the name of Jesus." Now that's a pretty good prayer compared to where she had come from, but I knew that it wouldn't work. Knowing that the burning hadn't left, I asked her, "Do you still have any burning?"

"Yes. Why didn't it leave?"

"Because you spoke to God about your burning instead of speaking to your burning." Then I opened my Bible to Mark 11:23 and shared more about this truth with her, saying, "You need to speak to your mountain."

She looked at me and said, "You mean I'm supposed to speak to burning—call it by that name, and actually speak to it?"

"Yes. That's what the Bible says to do."

You may think this is strange, but Jesus spoke to a fig tree. (see Mark 11:12–26.) He's the One who told us to speak to the mountain. (Mark 11:23.) It works. It's a law in His kingdom. You don't have to fully understand it to do it. When you flip a switch on the wall, you don't have to understand why your lights come on. You just do it, and it works. Release your faith and exercise your God-given authority by speaking to the mountain. It'll work.

So this woman prayed again, saying, "Burning, in the name of Jesus..." Immediately she stopped and exclaimed, "It's already gone!" That's all she had to say. God had set her free. I had dinner with her over a year later, and she was still walking in divine health. It was a great miracle!

One of the important keys I use is my words. Specifically, I don't just speak positive words to God, but I speak positive words to my situation. I take authority and command the situation to change. These are some of the laws of the kingdom. It may seem strange at first, but that's just how the kingdom works.

Receive It by Faith

If you have a financial problem, speak to your checkbook. Your checkbook is speaking to you, saying, "Look at all this red, and hardly any black. The Word didn't work. God isn't supplying your needs." You'll have those thoughts come to you as you look at your checkbook. So speak to the mountain. Say, "In the name of Jesus, my God supplies all of my needs according to His riches in glory by Christ Jesus. (Philippians 4:19.) I command this red ink to leave, and black ink to come. I call God's abundant provision into manifestation. My accounts receive money and increase."

Concerning physical healing, speak to your body. I recently rebuked sugar diabetes in a man at one of my meetings. I didn't ask God to rebuke it, I did. The Lord has already done His part. God had already healed this man. It's just a matter of someone here on earth releasing their faith by taking authority and speaking to the mountain.

There is so much more I could share with you about taking your authority and speaking to the mountain. It's really important that you receive this revelation and begin to walk in it. That's why I would like to recommend to you three of my teachings entitled *The Believer's Authority, You've Already Got It!* and *Spiritual Authority*. You have to learn that God has already done His part and now you must take your authority and command it to come to pass. Everything that Christ has provided through His death, burial, and resurrection is available right now in the spirit realm by grace, but in order for you to experience the manifestation of that provision in the physical realm you must reach out and receive it by faith.

Repair and Restore

I commanded this man's sugar diabetes to be gone. Then I spoke to his pancreas telling it to come back to life and begin to function properly. I did this because that was the part of his body that wasn't working properly. I commanded his insulin to come to a proper level, and so forth.

A month later, this guy came to me with an awesome report. He started clicking through the days of stored data in his electronic monitor that he used to test his blood sugar levels. I'm not exactly sure what it means, but his sugar level was up over 1,100 on the day that I prayed for him. Then it just started going down, and down, and down. He kept clicking through the data and showing me that every day it decreased. He was down to something like 108 at that time. This positive turnaround took place because I not only rebuked and commanded sugar diabetes to leave, but I also spoke to his body to repair.

I've actually had my hands on people with tumors that instantly left—right under my hand—when I prayed and rebuked cancer. I could feel the tumor go down. But I've also realized that diseases like that damage the body, so I'll speak to the parts of the body that were affected and release God's healing power.

I'll command the organs that were eaten away to re-grow and be restored. This is how I speak to the mountain.

When I pray for people with something like arthritis, I'll rebuke arthritis by name. I believe arthritis is a demonic spirit, so I'll rebuke the spirit and command arthritis to go in Jesus' name. If I were to stop there, they could be healed of arthritis, but the damage it caused in their body would still be there. So I not only rebuke arthritis, but I speak to the body to repair. I command twisted limbs to come back into proper placement. I command pain, swelling, and inflammation to be gone. I've seen the good results that come from cooperating with this spiritual law thousands of times.

The bottom line is, you must speak. The woman with the issue of blood spoke and said, "If I may but touch His clothes I'll be made whole." Then she acted on what she believed. It would have done her no good whatsoever to say what she said if she hadn't followed through with actions.

Chapter 18

Act On Your Faith

Faith without corresponding actions is dead.

> *But wilt thou know, O vain man, that faith without works is dead?*
>
> *James 2:20*

You must act on your faith. If you're sick but after you're through reading this book you start saying, "I believe in the name of Jesus I am healed," but then you continue to think sick, talk sick, and act sick, you won't see the manifestation of your healing. You need to meditate on God's Word concerning healing, speak it forth again and again until faith comes, and then act on your faith. If you've been lying in bed because you don't feel good, get up and start doing something. Move around. Begin acting on your faith.

Made Complete

I could share with you hundreds of examples of this truth in action. I've hurt my back before and suffered from excruciating pain. I didn't feel like moving, but I got up by faith and started doing exercises and sit-ups. I did everything I didn't feel like doing, resisting the pain. (James 4:7.) That was over thirty years ago. Praise God, I still have a strong and healthy back. But before I received the manifestation of healing, my back was in a very serious condition.

Another time I felt sick while working on a painting job. I came home for a lunch break and lay down on the couch, wanting to just do nothing. My wife, being the woman of faith that she is, got me up, put my arm around her neck, and made me dance with her through the house acting like I was healed. Within thirty minutes I was over it, went back to my painting job, and got paid that day (we really needed the money then).

Many people will lie in bed drinking sodas and popping pills. They'll let a loved one rub their fevered brow and wonder why they're still sick. Faith is perfected, made complete, by works.

> *Seest thou how faith wrought with his works, and by works was faith made perfect?*
>
> *James 2:22*

Now, don't misunderstand this truth by thinking that actions produce faith. They don't, and this is where many people have missed it. Some folks who weren't believing God, thought, *If I just act like I'm believing God, then it'll work.* So they quit taking their insulin, treatments, and medicine, and they died. Then faith gets a bad name. Works—actions—don't produce faith, but if you already have faith, then it won't be complete until you act on it.

Act on Your Faith

Focus and Commitment

The woman with the issue of blood had to act on what she believed. By faith, she had spoken, "If I may but touch His clothes, I shall be made whole." So she acted on that by working her way through the multitude of people thronging Jesus until she could reach out and touch the hem of His garment.

There's was no easy way for someone to reach down and touch the hem of a garment that was all the way down to the ground. That means this woman probably crawled on her hands and knees, aggressively pushing her way through this crowd of people surrounding Jesus. Her actions show complete commitment on her part.

According to the Old Testament law, her issue of blood made her unclean. Any garment or person she rubbed up against became unclean too. This was considered to be very offensive. People like her, with issues of blood, could not go out in public. If they did, they had to stand on the street corner and yell, "Unclean, unclean." People would then clear out of the way and give them a wide path to go through. By crawling and pushing her way through this crowd in order to touch Jesus' clothes, this woman was taking some serious risks. If it was discovered that she had an issue of blood, she could have been stoned to death. She wasn't going to let anything or anyone deter or stop her from receiving from God.

This illustrates another important law of the kingdom: *It takes focus and commitment to receive from God.*

161

God Wants You Well

"With All Your Heart"

Many people are very familiar with Jeremiah 29:11, which says:

For I know the thoughts that I think toward you, saith the LORD, thoughts of peace, and not of evil, to give you an expected end.

But they're not as familiar with verses 12 and 13, which continue the thought, saying:

Then shall ye call upon me, and ye shall go and pray unto me, and I will hearken unto you. And ye shall seek me, and find me, when ye shall search for me with all your heart.

Notice how God's Word here reveals that you'll search for Him and find Him when you search for Him with all of your heart. Many people passively pray, "God, I'd like to be healed," but in their heart, they could still live without it. They aren't committed to the point where they're saying, "I can't live without it." Because of that, they don't see the healing power of God manifest.

As long as you can live without being healed, you will. But when you reach a place where you say in your heart, "I am not going to take this anymore"; when you get the same amount of commitment that this woman with the issue of blood had that you are literally putting your life on the line because you could be trampled or stoned to death by the crowd; when you get focused and serious enough that you'll do whatever it takes to act on what you believe; when you get that kind of attitude, the power of God will begin to flow. That's just another law that governs how faith works.

A Clean Heart

Just like unbelief, unforgiveness can short-circuit the power of God.

> *His lord was wroth, and delivered him to the tormentors, till he should pay all that was due unto him. So likewise shall my heavenly Father do also unto you, if ye from your hearts forgive not every one his brother their trespasses.*
> *Matthew 18:34,35*

If you harbor unforgiveness in your heart, you'll be turned over to the tormentors. A root of bitterness will spring up and defile your entire body.

> *Looking diligently lest any man fail of the grace of God; lest any root of bitterness springing up trouble you, and thereby many be defiled.*
> *Hebrews 12:15*

You need to have a clean heart—a heart that's free from unforgiveness and bitterness.

How Faith Works

Also, faith works by love.

> *In Jesus Christ neither circumcision availeth any thing, nor uncircumcision; but faith which worketh by love.*
> *Galatians 5:6*

163

If you really understood how much God loves you, your faith would go through the roof. My teachings entitled *God's Kind of Love: The Cure for What Ails Ya* and *God's Love to You* would really help you understand the love and mercy of God. If you've been confused because of the wrath and punishment in the Old Testament, my teachings called *The True Nature of God* and *The War Is Over* would really open your eyes. When you understand how much God loves you, your faith will work.

A man and his twelve-year-old daughter came to one of my services. She was in a wheelchair and, basically, a vegetable. She was alive and breathing, but she couldn't communicate. Her mind wasn't working and her body didn't function. At twelve years of age, she was still using diapers. During the service, I said something about it being God's will to heal every time. This father became offended, and left. But the person who had brought him to the service convinced him to stick around until after the service saying, "Perhaps you misunderstood what Andrew said. Maybe he can explain himself." So he stayed, but he was mad at me.

I told him, "It's God's will to heal your daughter."

He answered, "God made my daughter this way. It's His will." I understood why he said that. It was a defense mechanism. It grieved him to see his daughter in that condition. I'm sure he had prayed, but he didn't see any results. So he just assumed that it was God's will, and that the Lord had some plan for his daughter to be like that.

"God Is Love"

I began to teach him from the scripture that this wasn't true. Well, he threw scriptures back at me justifying his position. I thought he was misinterpreting his scriptures, and he thought I was misinterpreting mine. We were at a standstill, and this man was very angry.

He was standing behind his daughter at the back of the wheelchair, and she was in between us. I was desperate to get this man to understand that God wanted his daughter healed, and I figured I had nothing to lose since he was already mad at me. So finally, I just laid into him, saying, "What kind of a father are you, anyway? What kind of a father wants his daughter to be a quadriplegic, a vegetable, bound to a wheelchair all her life? She'll never get to play, get married, or have any other joys in life. What kind of a man are you?"

This guy was already hot, but the steam just started shooting out of his ears. He could have beat me up, and I'm sure he considered it, but he looked at me with rage in his eyes, and answered, "I would do anything to help my daughter get well. If there was an operation, I would spend any amount of money. If I could take her place and become like her so that she could be normal, I would do it. I'd do anything to get her healed!"

After he spouted all that, I looked him straight in the eye, saying, "And you think God—who has all power—loves your daughter less than you do."

That stopped him stone cold. He had a doctrine and an argument. He'd been taught wrong that God puts sickness and

165

disease on people. He loved his daughter, and would have done anything for her. There were no lengths he wouldn't go to, to produce healing. So I turned the tables and challenged him saying, "You think God—who the Bible says is love—loves your daughter less than you do." He could argue doctrine, but not when I brought it down to love.

God is love.

1 John 4:8

If you really understood and believed how much God loves you, your faith would shoot through the roof believing that God is healing you. It's not the Lord who hasn't healed, it's us who haven't understood and received. We need to understand how much God loves us. We need to focus and meditate on His love for us. That alone would work wonders for our faith.

The Owner's Manual

You may be insistent and focused on healing, but you don't understand how much God loves you. You might think He's upset. You may hate yourself. You may be disappointed with yourself, and think the Lord dislikes you even more. That is a big hindrance to God's healing power flowing in your life. Remember that faith works by love. (Galatians 5:6.) It's another kingdom law. So if you want to see the Lord's healing power manifest in your life, you need to start understanding how much He loves you.

On and on we could go. I've discovered many more laws like this that govern how faith works.

I've only been able to share a few of the most important ones in this book. Personally, I still don't understand all there is to know about faith and healing, but it's all revealed in the Word of God.

God's Word is the owner's manual. As born-again believers, we belong to Him, and His Word tells us how His kingdom works. We need to get into His word and discover more of the laws that govern how faith works. Then, by faith, we need to cooperate with those laws.

Consider different people in the Bible and how they received their healing. Meditate (ponder or think) on the woman with the issue of blood. Study Jairus who received his daughter back from the dead. Look at how Jesus ministered healing to others. Pray and ask the Holy Spirit to help you see things that would apply to you and to the people to whom He wants you to minister healing.

God wants you well. He wants you well more than you want to be well. If you aren't well, it's not because God isn't willing. It's because you haven't understood how to receive. There's something you're doing in your life, probably some of the things we've discussed in this book, that's hindering you. Maybe you've been speaking forth negative things. You've been complaining, murmuring, and saying what the doctor had to say instead of what God has to say. Perhaps you're more moved by your medical report than by God's report in the Scriptures. You need to start declaring what God says in His Word.

You need to speak to your mountain—directly to your problem. You need to act on your faith. You need to understand the love of God, and start walking in forgiveness. Get committed enough that nothing will deter you from receiving by faith what God has supplied. As long as you can live without being healed, you will. But once you are determined that you're not going to live like this any longer, it'll make a difference.

My Prayer for
Your Healing

God is a good God. He's already provided everything you need, including healing. God wants you well. He is for you. If you'll let Him, He will guide you into all truth and show you what you need to do to be able to receive your healing.

I want to pray for you now.

Father, I pray for my friend reading this book right now. I know it's Your will for them to be well. I know that You've already done it, for by Your stripes they have already been healed. (1 Peter 2:24.) Lord, You've already generated the power. It's there. We just need to flip the switch. It's just a matter of learning and changing our thinking. Father, I pray that right now the Holy Spirit would quicken on the inside of my friend whatever it is that they need to change so that they can receive what You've already done.

Your Word says that all things that pertain to life and godliness are given to us through the knowledge of Him. (2 Peter 1:3.) Father, I ask You to impart to my friend the knowledge they need right now to release and experience Your healing power.

We speak to this problem now, in the name of Jesus. We command any kind of tumors, cancer, or anything else that has invaded their body to die. Germs, viruses, infections, and the like, die in the name of Jesus. Father, we loose Your anointing to flow through their body to release them from pain and all these other symptoms. We go to the root of the problem and command these things to be healed.

In Jesus' name, I command fear to be gone, faith to come, and love to flow. We agree with You that we were healed, and if we were (past tense) healed, then we are (present tense) healed. Father, we thank You that You want us well. We receive that in Jesus' name. Amen.

Is It Always God's
Will to Heal?

There are seventeen times in the Gospels where Jesus healed all of the sick who were present. There are forty-seven other times where He healed one or two people at a time. Nowhere do we find the Lord refusing to heal anyone.

In fact, Jesus declared that He could do nothing of Himself but only what He saw the Father do.

> *Then answered Jesus and said unto them, Verily, verily, I say unto you, The Son can do nothing of himself, but what he seeth the Father do: for what things soever he doeth, these also doeth the Son likewise.*
>
> *John 5:19*

> *Then said Jesus unto them, When ye have lifted up the Son of man, then shall ye know that I am he, and that I do nothing of myself; but as my Father hath taught me, I speak these things. And he that sent me is with me: the Father hath not left me alone; for I do always those things that please him.*
>
> *John 8:28,29*

In light of these statements, Jesus' actions are proof enough that it is always God's will to heal!

Scriptures

Seventeen times in the Gospels Jesus healed all of the sick who were present:

1. Jesus went about all Galilee, teaching in their synagogues, and preaching the gospel of the kingdom, and healing all manner of sickness and all manner of disease among the people. And his fame went throughout all Syria: and they brought unto him all sick people that were taken with divers diseases and torments, and those which were possessed with devils, and those which were lunatic, and those that had the palsy; and he healed them.

Matthew 4:23,24

2. When the even was come, they brought unto him many that were possessed with devils: and he cast out the spirits with his word, and healed all that were sick: That it might be fulfilled which was spoken by Esaias the prophet, saying, Himself took our infirmities, and bare our sicknesses.

Matthew 8:16,17

3. Jesus went about all the cities and villages, teaching in their synagogues, and preaching the gospel of the kingdom, and healing every sickness and every disease among the people.

Matthew 9:35

4. When Jesus knew it, he withdrew himself from thence: and great multitudes followed him, and he healed them all.

Matthew 12:15

5. Jesus went forth, and saw a great multitude, and was moved with compassion toward them, and he healed their sick.

Matthew 14:14

6. When they were gone over, they came into the land of Gennesaret. And when the men of that place had knowledge of him, they sent out into all that country round about, and brought unto him all that were diseased; And besought him that they might only touch the hem of his garment: and as many as touched were made perfectly whole.

Matthew 14:34–36

7. Great multitudes came unto him, having with them those that were lame, blind, dumb, maimed, and many others, and cast them down at Jesus' feet; and he healed them: Insomuch that the multitude wondered, when they saw the dumb to speak, the maimed to be whole, the lame to walk, and the blind to see: and they glorified the God of Israel.

Matthew 15:30,31

8. Great multitudes followed him; and he healed them there.

Matthew 19:2

9. The blind and the lame came to him in the temple; and he healed them.

Matthew 21:14

10. At even, when the sun did set, they brought unto him all that were diseased, and them that were possessed with devils.

And all the city was gathered together at the door. And he healed many that were sick of divers diseases, and cast out many devils; and suffered not the devils to speak, because they knew him.

Mark 1:32–34

11. He preached in their synagogues throughout all Galilee, and cast out devils.

Mark 1:39

12. Whithersoever he entered, into villages, or cities, or country, they laid the sick in the streets, and besought him that they might touch if it were but the border of his garment: and as many as touched him were made whole.

Mark 6:56

13. Now when the sun was setting, all they that had any sick with divers diseases brought them unto him; and he laid his hands on every one of them, and healed them.

Luke 4:40

14. He came down with them, and stood in the plain, and the company of his disciples, and a great multitude of people out of all Judaea and Jerusalem, and from the sea coast of Tyre and Sidon, which came to hear him, and to be healed of their diseases; And they that were vexed with unclean spirits: and they were healed. And the whole multitude sought to touch him: for there went virtue out of him, and healed them all.

Luke 6:17–19

15. In that same hour he cured many of their infirmities and plagues, and of evil spirits; and unto many that were blind he gave sight.

Luke 7:21

16. The people, when they knew it, followed him: and he received them, and spake unto them of the kingdom of God, and healed them that had need of healing.

Luke 9:11

17. As he entered into a certain village, there met him ten men that were lepers, which stood afar off: And they lifted up their voices, and said, Jesus, Master, have mercy on us. And when he saw them, he said unto them, Go show yourselves unto the priests. And it came to pass, that, as they went, they were cleansed. And one of them, when he saw that he was healed, turned back, and with a loud voice glorified God, And fell down on his face at his feet, giving him thanks: and he was a Samaritan. And Jesus answering said, Were there not ten cleansed? but where are the nine?

Luke 17:12–17

Forty-seven other times, the Gospels show Jesus healed one or two people at a time:

1. When he was come down from the mountain, great multitudes followed him. And, behold, there came a leper and worshipped him, saying, Lord, if thou wilt, thou canst make me clean. And Jesus put forth his hand, and touched him, saying, I will; be thou clean. And immediately his leprosy was cleansed. And Jesus saith unto him, See thou tell no man; but go thy way, show thyself to the priest, and offer the gift that Moses commanded, for a testimony unto them.

Matthew 8:1–4

2. When Jesus was entered into Capernaum, there came unto him a centurion, beseeching him, And saying, Lord, my servant lieth at home sick of the palsy, grievously tormented. And Jesus saith unto him, I will come and heal him. The centurion answered and said, Lord, I am not worthy that thou shouldest come under my roof: but speak the word only, and my servant shall be healed. For I am a man under authority, having soldiers under me: and I say to this man, Go, and he goeth; and to another, Come, and he cometh; and to my servant, Do this, and he doeth it. When Jesus heard it, he marvelled, and said to them that followed, Verily I say unto you, I have not found so great faith, no, not in Israel. And I say unto you, That many shall come from the east and west, and shall sit down with Abraham, and Isaac, and Jacob, in the kingdom of heaven. But the children of the kingdom shall be cast out into outer darkness: there shall be weeping and gnashing of teeth. And Jesus said unto the centurion, Go thy way; and as thou hast

believed, so be it done unto thee. And his servant was healed
in the selfsame hour.

Matthew 8:5–13

3. When Jesus was come into Peter's house, he saw his wife's
mother laid, and sick of a fever. And he touched her hand, and
the fever left her: and she arose, and ministered unto them.

Matthew 8:14–15

4. When he was come to the other side into the country of the
Gergesenes, there met him two possessed with devils, coming
out of the tombs, exceeding fierce, so that no man might pass by
that way. And, behold, they cried out, saying, What have we to
do with thee, Jesus, thou Son of God? art thou come hither to
torment us before the time? And there was a good way off from
them an herd of many swine feeding. So the devils besought
him, saying, If thou cast us out, suffer us to go away into the
herd of swine. And he said unto them, Go. And when they were
come out, they went into the herd of swine: and, behold, the
whole herd of swine ran violently down a steep place into the
sea, and perished in the waters. And they that kept them fled,
and went their ways into the city, and told every thing, and
what was befallen to the possessed of the devils. And, behold,
the whole city came out to meet Jesus: and when they saw him,
they besought him that he would depart out of their coasts.

Matthew 8:28–34

5. He entered into a ship, and passed over, and came into his
own city. And, behold, they brought to him a man sick of the

palsy, lying on a bed: and Jesus seeing their faith said unto the sick of the palsy; Son, be of good cheer; thy sins be forgiven thee. And, behold, certain of the scribes said within themselves, This man blasphemeth. And Jesus knowing their thoughts said, Wherefore think ye evil in your hearts? For whether is easier, to say, Thy sins be forgiven thee; or to say, Arise, and walk? But that ye may know that the Son of man hath power on earth to forgive sins, (then saith he to the sick of the palsy,) Arise, take up thy bed, and go unto thine house. And he arose, and departed to his house. But when the multitudes saw it, they marvelled, and glorified God, which had given such power unto men.

Matthew 9:1–8

6. And, behold, a woman, which was diseased with an issue of blood twelve years, came behind him, and touched the hem of his garment: For she said within herself, If I may but touch his garment, I shall be whole. But Jesus turned him about, and when he saw her, he said, Daughter, be of good comfort; thy faith hath made thee whole. And the woman was made whole from that hour.

Matthew 9:20–22

7. When Jesus came into the ruler's house, and saw the minstrels and the people making a noise, He said unto them, Give place: for the maid is not dead, but sleepeth. And they laughed him to scorn. But when the people were put forth, he went in, and took her by the hand, and the maid arose. And the fame hereof went abroad into all that land.

Matthew 9:23–26

8. When Jesus departed thence, two blind men followed him, crying, and saying, Thou Son of David, have mercy on us. And when he was come into the house, the blind men came to him: and Jesus saith unto them, Believe ye that I am able to do this? They said unto him, Yea, Lord. Then touched he their eyes, saying, According to your faith be it unto you. And their eyes were opened; and Jesus straitly charged them, saying, See that no man know it. But they, when they were departed, spread abroad his fame in all that country.

Matthew 9:27–31

9. As they went out, behold, they brought to him a dumb man possessed with a devil. And when the devil was cast out, the dumb spake: and the multitudes marvelled, saying, It was never so seen in Israel.

Matthew 9:32–33

10. And, behold, there was a man which had his hand withered. And they asked him, saying, Is it lawful to heal on the sabbath days? that they might accuse him. And he said unto them, What man shall there be among you, that shall have one sheep, and if it fall into a pit on the sabbath day, will he not lay hold on it, and lift it out? How much then is a man better than a sheep? Wherefore it is lawful to do well on the sabbath days. Then saith he to the man, Stretch forth thine hand. And he stretched it forth; and it was restored whole, like as the other.

Matthew 12:10–13

11. Then was brought unto him one possessed with a devil, blind, and dumb: and he healed him, insomuch that the blind and dumb both spake and saw. And all the people were amazed, and said, Is not this the son of David?

Matthew 12:22–23

12. Then Jesus went thence, and departed into the coasts of Tyre and Sidon. And, behold, a woman of Canaan came out of the same coasts, and cried unto him, saying, Have mercy on me, O Lord, thou Son of David; my daughter is grievously vexed with a devil. But he answered her not a word. And his disciples came and besought him, saying, Send her away; for she crieth after us. But he answered and said, I am not sent but unto the lost sheep of the house of Israel. Then came she and worshipped him, saying, Lord, help me. But he answered and said, It is not meet to take the children's bread, and to cast it to dogs. And she said, Truth, Lord: yet the dogs eat of the crumbs which fall from their masters' table. Then Jesus answered and said unto her, O woman, great is thy faith: be it unto thee even as thou wilt. And her daughter was made whole from that very hour.

Matthew 15:21–28

13. When they were come to the multitude, there came to him a certain man, kneeling down to him, and saying, Lord, have mercy on my son: for he is lunatic, and sore vexed: for ofttimes he falleth into the fire, and oft into the water. And I brought him to thy disciples, and they could not cure him. Then Jesus answered and said, O faithless and perverse generation, how long shall I be with you? how long shall I suffer you? bring him hither to me. And Jesus rebuked the devil; and he departed out of him: and the child was cured from that very hour.

Matthew 17:14–18

181

14. And, behold, two blind men sitting by the way side, when they heard that Jesus passed by, cried out, saying, Have mercy on us, O Lord, thou Son of David. And the multitude rebuked them, because they should hold their peace: but they cried the more, saying, Have mercy on us, O Lord, thou Son of David. And Jesus stood still, and called them, and said, What will ye that I shall do unto you? They say unto him, Lord, that our eyes may be opened. So Jesus had compassion on them, and touched their eyes: and immediately their eyes received sight, and they followed him.

Matthew 20:30–34

15. They went into Capernaum; and straightway on the sabbath day he entered into the synagogue, and taught. And they were astonished at his doctrine: for he taught them as one that had authority, and not as the scribes. And there was in their synagogue a man with an unclean spirit; and he cried out, Saying, Let us alone; what have we to do with thee, thou Jesus of Nazareth? art thou come to destroy us? I know thee who thou art, the Holy One of God. And Jesus rebuked him, saying, Hold thy peace, and come out of him. And when the unclean spirit had torn him, and cried with a loud voice, he came out of him. And they were all amazed, insomuch that they questioned among themselves, saying, What thing is this? what new doctrine is this? for with authority commandeth he even the unclean spirits, and they do obey him. And immediately his fame spread abroad throughout all the region round about Galilee.

Mark 1:21–28

16. *Forthwith, when they were come out of the synagogue,*
they entered into the house of Simon and Andrew, with James
and John. But Simon's wife's mother lay sick of a fever, and
anon they tell him of her. And he came and took her by the
hand, and lifted her up; and immediately the fever left her,
and she ministered unto them.

Mark 1:29–31

17. *There came a leper to him, beseeching him, and kneeling*
down to him, and saying unto him, If thou wilt, thou canst
make me clean. And Jesus, moved with compassion, put
forth his hand, and touched him, and saith unto him, I will;
be thou clean. And as soon as he had spoken, immediately
the leprosy departed from him, and he was cleansed. And
he straitly charged him, and forthwith sent him away; And
saith unto him, See thou say nothing to any man: but go thy
way, show thyself to the priest, and offer for thy cleansing
those things which Moses commanded, for a testimony unto
them. But he went out, and began to publish it much, and
to blaze abroad the matter, insomuch that Jesus could no
more openly enter into the city, but was without in desert
places: and they came to him from every quarter.

Mark 1:40–45

18. *And again he entered into Capernaum after some days;*
and it was noised that he was in the house. And straightway
many were gathered together, insomuch that there was no
room to receive them, no, not so much as about the door: and
he preached the word unto them. And they come unto him,

bringing one sick of the palsy, which was borne of four. And when they could not come nigh unto him for the press, they uncovered the roof where he was: and when they had broken it up, they let down the bed wherein the sick of the palsy lay. When Jesus saw their faith, he said unto the sick of the palsy, Son, thy sins be forgiven thee. But there were certain of the scribes sitting there, and reasoning in their hearts, Why doth this man thus speak blasphemies? who can forgive sins but God only? And immediately when Jesus perceived in his spirit that

they so reasoned within themselves, he said unto them, Why reason ye these things in your hearts? Whether is it easier to say to the sick of the palsy, Thy sins be forgiven thee; or to say, Arise, and take up thy bed, and walk? But that ye may know that the Son of man hath power on earth to forgive sins, (he saith to the sick of the palsy,) I say unto thee, Arise, and take up thy bed, and go thy way into thine house. And immediately he arose, took up the bed, and went forth before them all; insomuch that they were all amazed, and glorified God, saying, We never saw it on this fashion.

Mark 2:1–12

19. He entered again into the synagogue; and there was a man there which had a withered hand. And they watched him, whether he would heal him on the sabbath day; that they might accuse him. And he saith unto the man which had the withered hand, Stand forth. And he saith unto them, Is it lawful to do good on the sabbath days, or to do evil? to save life, or to kill? But they held their peace. And when he had looked round about on them with anger, being grieved for

the hardness of their hearts, he saith unto the man, Stretch
forth thine hand. And he stretched it out: and his hand was
restored whole as the other.

Mark 3:1–5

20. *They came over unto the other side of the sea, into the*
country of the Gadarenes. And when he was come out of the
ship, immediately there met him out of the tombs a man with
an unclean spirit, Who had his dwelling among the tombs;
and no man could bind him, no, not with chains: Because
that he had been often bound with fetters and chains, and
the chains had been plucked asunder by him, and the fetters
broken in pieces: neither could any man tame him. And
always, night and day, he was in the mountains, and in the
tombs, crying, and cutting himself with stones. But when he
saw Jesus afar off, he ran and worshipped him, And cried
with a loud voice, and said, What have I to do with thee,
Jesus, thou Son of the most high God? I adjure thee by God,
that thou torment me not. For he said unto him, Come out
of the man, thou unclean spirit. And he asked him, What is
thy name? And he answered, saying, My name is Legion: for
we are many. And he besought him much that he would not
send them away out of the country. Now there was there nigh
unto the mountains a great herd of swine feeding. And all the
devils besought him, saying, Send us into the swine, that we
may enter into them. And forthwith Jesus gave them leave.
And the unclean spirits went out, and entered into the swine:
and the herd ran violently down a steep place into the sea,
(they were about two thousand;) and were choked in the sea.
And they that fed the swine fled, and told it in the city, and in

the country. And they went out to see what it was that was done. And they come to Jesus, and see him that was possessed with the devil, and had the legion, sitting, and clothed, and in his right mind: and they were afraid. And they that saw it told them how it befell to him that was possessed with the devil, and also concerning the swine. And they began to pray him to depart out of their coasts. And when he was come into the ship, he that had been possessed with the devil prayed him that he might be with him. Howbeit Jesus suffered him not, but saith unto him, Go home to thy friends, and tell them how great things the Lord hath done for thee, and hath had compassion on thee. And he departed, and began to publish in Decapolis how great things Jesus had done for him: and all men did marvel.

Mark 5:1–20

21. A certain woman, which had an issue of blood twelve years, And had suffered many things of many physicians, and had spent all that she had, and was nothing bettered, but rather grew worse, When she had heard of Jesus, came in the press behind, and touched his garment. For she said, If I may touch but his clothes, I shall be whole. And straightway the fountain of her blood was dried up; and she felt in her body that she was healed of that plague. And Jesus, immediately knowing in himself that virtue had gone out of him, turned him about in the press, and said, Who touched my clothes? And his disciples said unto him, Thou seest the multitude thronging thee, and sayest thou, Who touched me? And he looked round about to see her that had done this thing. But the woman fearing and trembling, knowing what was done

in her, came and fell down before him, and told him all the truth. And he said unto her, Daughter, thy faith hath made thee whole; go in peace, and be whole of thy plague.

Mark 5:25–34

22. *While he yet spake, there came from the ruler of the synagogue's house certain which said, Thy daughter is dead: why troublest thou the Master any further? As soon as Jesus heard the word that was spoken, he saith unto the ruler of the synagogue, Be not afraid, only believe. And he suffered no man to follow him, save Peter, and James, and John the brother of James. And he cometh to the house of the ruler of the synagogue, and seeth the tumult, and them that wept and wailed greatly. And when he was come in, he saith unto them, Why make ye this ado, and weep? the damsel is not dead, but sleepeth. And they laughed him to scorn. But when he had put them all out, he taketh the father and the mother of the damsel, and them that were with him, and entereth in where the damsel was lying. And he took the damsel by the hand, and said unto her, Talitha cumi; which is, being interpreted, Damsel, I say unto thee, arise. And straightway the damsel arose, and walked; for she was of the age of twelve years. And they were astonished with a great astonishment. And he charged them straitly that no man should know it; and commanded that something should be given her to eat.*

Mark 5:35–43

23. *From thence he arose, and went into the borders of Tyre and Sidon, and entered into an house, and would have no man know it: but he could not be hid. For a certain woman,*

whose young daughter had an unclean spirit, heard of him, and came and fell at his feet: The woman was a Greek, a Syrophenician by nation; and she besought him that he would cast forth the devil out of her daughter. But Jesus said unto her, Let the children first be filled: for it is not meet to take the children's bread, and to cast it unto the dogs. And she answered and said unto him, Yes, Lord: yet the dogs under the table eat of the children's crumbs. And he said unto her, For this saying go thy way; the devil is gone out of thy daughter. And when she was come to her house, she found the devil gone out, and her daughter laid upon the bed.

Mark 7:24–30

24. And again, departing from the coasts of Tyre and Sidon, he came unto the sea of Galilee, through the midst of the coasts of Decapolis. And they bring unto him one that was deaf, and had an impediment in his speech; and they beseech him to put his hand upon him. And he took him aside from the multitude, and put his fingers into his ears, and he spit, and touched his tongue; And looking up to heaven, he sighed, and saith unto him, Ephphatha, that is, Be opened. And straightway his ears were opened, and the string of his tongue was loosed, and he spake plain. And he charged them that they should tell no man: but the more he charged them, so much the more a great deal they published it; And were beyond measure astonished, saying, He hath done all things well: he maketh both the deaf to hear, and the dumb to speak.

Mark 7:31–37

25. He cometh to Bethsaida; and they bring a blind man unto him, and besought him to touch him. And he took the blind man by the hand, and led him out of the town; and when he had spit on his eyes, and put his hands upon him, he asked him if he saw ought. And he looked up, and said, I see men as trees, walking. After that he put his hands again upon his eyes, and made him look up: and he was restored, and saw every man clearly. And he sent him away to his house, saying, Neither go into the town, nor tell it to any in the town.

Mark 8:22–26

26. *When he came to his disciples, he saw a great multitude about them, and the scribes questioning with them. And straightway all the people, when they beheld him, were greatly amazed, and running to him saluted him. And he asked the scribes, What question ye with them? And one of the multitude answered and said, Master, I have brought unto thee my son, which hath a dumb spirit; And wheresoever he taketh him, he teareth him: and he foameth, and gnasheth with his teeth, and pineth away: and I spake to thy disciples that they should cast him out; and they could not. He answereth him, and saith, O faithless generation, how long shall I be with you? how long shall I suffer you? bring him unto me. And they brought him unto him: and when he saw him, straightway the spirit tare him; and he fell on the ground, and wallowed foaming. And he asked his father, How long is it ago since this came unto him? And he said, Of a child. And ofttimes it hath cast him into the fire, and into the waters, to destroy him: but if thou canst do any thing, have compassion on us, and help us. Jesus said unto him, If thou canst believe, all things are possible to him that believeth. And straightway the father of the child cried out, and said with tears, Lord, I believe; help thou mine unbelief.*

189

When Jesus saw that the people came running together, he rebuked the foul spirit, saying unto him, Thou dumb and deaf spirit, I charge thee, come out of him, and enter no more into him. And the spirit cried, and rent him sore, and came out of him: and he was as one dead; insomuch that many said, He is dead. But Jesus took him by the hand, and lifted him up; and he arose. And when he was come into the house, his disciples asked him privately, Why could not we cast him out? And he said unto them, This kind can come forth by nothing, but by prayer and fasting.

Mark 9:14–29

27. They came to Jericho: and as he went out of Jericho with his disciples and a great number of people, blind Bartimaeus, the son of Timaeus, sat by the highway side begging. And when he heard that it was Jesus of Nazareth, he began to cry out, and say, Jesus, thou Son of David, have mercy on me. And many charged him that he should hold his peace: but he cried the more a great deal, Thou Son of David, have mercy on me. And Jesus stood still, and commanded him to be called. And they call the blind man, saying unto him, Be of good comfort, rise; he calleth thee. And he, casting away his garment, rose, and came to Jesus. And Jesus answered and said unto him, What wilt thou that I should do unto thee? The blind man said unto him, Lord, that I might receive my sight. And Jesus said unto him, Go thy way; thy faith hath made thee whole. And immediately he received his sight, and followed Jesus in the way.

Mark 10:46–52

190

28. In the synagogue there was a man, which had a spirit of an unclean devil, and cried out with a loud voice, Saying, Let us alone; what have we to do with thee, thou Jesus of Nazareth? art thou come to destroy us? I know thee who thou art; the Holy One of God. And Jesus rebuked him, saying, Hold thy peace, and come out of him. And when the devil had thrown him in the midst, he came out of him, and hurt him not. And they were all amazed, and spake among themselves, saying, What a word is this! for with authority and power he commandeth the unclean spirits, and they come out. And the fame of him went out into every place of the country round about. Luke 4:33–37

29. He arose out of the synagogue, and entered into Simon's house. And Simon's wife's mother was taken with a great fever; and they besought him for her. And he stood over her, and rebuked the fever; and it left her: and immediately she arose and ministered unto them.

Luke 4:38–39

30. It came to pass, when he was in a certain city, behold a man full of leprosy: who seeing Jesus fell on his face, and besought him, saying, Lord, if thou wilt, thou canst make me clean. And he put forth his hand, and touched him, saying, I will: be thou clean. And immediately the leprosy departed from him. And he charged him to tell no man: but go, and show thyself to the priest, and offer for thy cleansing, according as Moses commanded, for a testimony unto them. But so much the more went there a fame abroad of him: and great multitudes came together to hear, and to be healed by him of their infirmities.

Luke 5:12–15

31. It came to pass on a certain day, as he was teaching, that there were Pharisees and doctors of the law sitting by, which were come out of every town of Galilee, and Judaea, and Jerusalem: and the power of the Lord was present to heal them. And, behold, men brought in a bed a man which was taken with a palsy: and they sought means to bring him in, and to lay him before him. And when they could not find by what way they might bring him in because of the multitude, they went upon the housetop, and let him down through the tiling with his couch into the midst before Jesus. And when he saw their faith, he said unto him, Man, thy sins are forgiven thee. And the scribes and the Pharisees began to reason, saying, Who is this which speaketh blasphemies? Who can forgive sins, but God alone? But when Jesus perceived their thoughts, he answering said unto them, What reason ye in your hearts? Whether is easier, to say, Thy sins be forgiven thee; or to say, Rise up and walk? But that ye may know that the Son of man hath power upon earth to forgive sins, (he said unto the sick of the palsy,) I say unto thee, Arise, and take up thy couch, and go into thine house. And immediately he rose up before them, and took up that whereon he lay, and departed to his own house, glorifying God. And they were all amazed, and they glorified God, and were filled with fear, saying, We have seen strange things to day.

Luke 5:17–26

32. It came to pass also on another sabbath, that he entered into the synagogue and taught: and there was a man whose right hand was withered. And the scribes and Pharisees watched him, whether he would heal on the sabbath day; that they might find an accusation against him. But he knew their thoughts, and said to the man which had the withered hand, Rise up, and stand forth in the midst. And he arose and stood forth. Then said Jesus unto them, I will ask you one thing; Is it lawful on the sabbath days to do good, or to do evil? to save life, or to destroy it? And looking round about upon them all, he said unto the man, Stretch forth thy hand. And he did so: and his hand was restored whole as the other.

Luke 6:6–10

33. Now when he had ended all his sayings in the audience of the people, he entered into Capernaum. And a certain centurion's servant, who was dear unto him, was sick, and ready to die. And when he heard of Jesus, he sent unto him the elders of the Jews, beseeching him that he would come and heal his servant. And when they came to Jesus, they besought him instantly, saying, That he was worthy for whom he should do this: For he loveth our nation, and he hath built us a synagogue. Then Jesus went with them. And when he was now not far from the house, the centurion sent friends to him, saying unto him, Lord, trouble not thyself: for I am not worthy that thou shouldest enter under my roof: Wherefore neither thought I myself worthy to come unto thee: but say in a word, and my servant shall be healed. For I also am a man set under authority, having under me soldiers, and I say unto one, Go, and he goeth; and to another, Come, and he cometh; and to my servant, Do this, and he doeth it. When Jesus heard these things, he marvelled at him, and turned him about, and said unto the people that followed him, I say unto you, I have not found so great faith, no, not in Israel. And they that were sent, returning to the house, found the servant whole that had been sick.

Luke 7:1–10

34. And it came to pass the day after, that he went into a city called Nain; and many of his disciples went with him, and much people. Now when he came nigh to the gate of the city, behold, there was a dead man carried out, the only son of his mother, and she was a widow: and much people of the city was with her. And when the Lord saw her, he had compassion on her, and said unto her, Weep not. And he came and touched the bier: and they that bare him stood still. And he said, Young man, I say unto thee, Arise. And he that was dead sat up, and began to speak. And he delivered him to his mother. And there came a fear on all: and they glorified God, saying, That a great prophet is risen up among us; and, That God hath visited his people. And this rumour of him went forth throughout all Judaea, and throughout all the region round about.

Luke 7:11–17

35. When he went forth to land, there met him out of the city a certain man, which had devils long time, and ware no clothes, neither abode in any house, but in the tombs. When he

saw Jesus, he cried out, and fell down before him, and with a
loud voice said, What have I to do with thee, Jesus, thou Son
of God most high? I beseech thee, torment me not. (For he had
commanded the unclean spirit to come out of the man. For
oftentimes it had caught him: and he was kept bound with
chains and in fetters; and he brake the bands, and was driven
of the devil into the wilderness.) And Jesus asked him, saying,
What is thy name? And he said, Legion: because many devils
were entered into him. And they besought him that he would
not command them to go out into the deep. And there was
there an herd of many swine feeding on the mountain: and
they besought him that he would suffer them to enter into
them. And he suffered them. Then went the devils out of the
man, and entered into the swine: and the herd ran violently
down a steep place into the lake, and were choked. When they
that fed them saw what was done, they fled, and went and
told it in the city and in the country. Then they went out to
see what was done; and came to Jesus, and found the man,
out of whom the devils were departed, sitting at the feet of
Jesus, clothed, and in his right mind: and they were afraid.
They also which saw it told them by what means he that was
possessed of the devils was healed. Then the whole multitude
of the country of the Gadarenes round about besought him to
depart from them; for they were taken with great fear: and
he went up into the ship, and returned back again. Now the
man out of whom the devils were departed besought him
that he might be with him: but Jesus sent him away, saying,
Return to thine own house, and show how great things God

hath done unto thee. And he went his way, and published throughout the whole city how great things Jesus had done unto him.

Luke 8:27–39

36. *A woman having an issue of blood twelve years, which had spent all her living upon physicians, neither could be healed of any, Came behind him, and touched the border of his garment: and immediately her issue of blood stanched. And Jesus said, Who touched me? When all denied, Peter and they that were with him said, Master, the multitude throng thee and press thee, and sayest thou, Who touched me? And Jesus said, Somebody hath touched me: for I perceive that virtue is gone out of me. And when the woman saw that she was not hid, she came trembling, and falling down before him, she declared unto him before all the people for what cause she had touched him, and how she was healed immediately. And he said unto her, Daughter, be of good comfort: thy faith hath made thee whole; go in peace.*

Luke 8:43–48

37. *While he yet spake, there cometh one from the ruler of the synagogue's house, saying to him, Thy daughter is dead; trouble not the Master. But when Jesus heard it, he answered him, saying, Fear not: believe only, and she shall be made whole. And when he came into the house, he suffered no man to go in, save Peter, and James, and John, and the father and the mother of the maiden. And all wept, and bewailed her: but he said, Weep not; she is not dead, but sleepeth. And*

they laughed him to scorn, knowing that she was dead. And he put them all out, and took her by the hand, and called, saying, Maid, arise. And her spirit came again, and she arose straightway: and he commanded to give her meat. And her parents were astonished: but he charged them that they should tell no man what was done.

Luke 8:49–56

38. It came to pass, that on the next day, when they were come down from the hill, much people met him. And, behold, a man of the company cried out, saying, Master, I beseech thee, look upon my son: for he is mine only child. And, lo, a spirit taketh him, and he suddenly crieth out; and it teareth him that he foameth again, and bruising him hardly departeth from him. And I besought thy disciples to cast him out; and they could not. And Jesus answering said, O faithless and perverse generation, how long shall I be with you, and suffer you? Bring thy son hither. And as he was yet a coming, the devil threw him down, and tare him. And Jesus rebuked the unclean spirit, and healed the child, and delivered him again to his father.

Luke 9:37–42

39. And he was casting out a devil, and it was dumb. And it came to pass, when the devil was gone out, the dumb spake; and the people wondered.

Luke 11:14

40. And, behold, there was a woman which had a spirit of infirmity eighteen years, and was bowed together, and could in no wise lift up herself. And when Jesus saw her, he called her to him, and said unto her, Woman, thou art loosed from thine infirmity. And he laid his hands on her: and immediately she was made straight, and glorified God. And the ruler of the synagogue answered with indignation, because that Jesus had healed on the sabbath day, and said unto the people, There are six days in which men ought to work: in them therefore come and be healed, and not on the sabbath day. The Lord then answered him, and said, Thou hypocrite, doth not each one of you on the sabbath loose his ox or his ass from the stall, and lead him away to watering? And ought not this woman, being a daughter of Abraham, whom Satan hath bound, lo, these eighteen years, be loosed from this bond on the sabbath day? And when he had said these things, all his adversaries were ashamed: and all the people rejoiced for all the glorious things that were done by him.

Luke 13:11–17

41. It came to pass, as he went into the house of one of the chief Pharisees to eat bread on the sabbath day, that they watched him. And, behold, there was a certain man before him which had the dropsy. And Jesus answering spake unto the lawyers and Pharisees, saying, Is it lawful to heal on the sabbath day? And they held their peace. And he took him, and healed him, and let him go; And answered them, saying, Which of you shall have an ass or an ox fallen into a pit, and will not straightway pull him out on the sabbath day?

Luke 14:1–5

42. It came to pass, that as he was come nigh unto Jericho, a certain blind man sat by the way side begging: And hearing the multitude pass by, he asked what it meant. And they told him, that Jesus of Nazareth passeth by. And he cried, saying, Jesus, thou Son of David, have mercy on me. And they which went before rebuked him, that he should hold his peace: but he cried so much the more, Thou Son of David, have mercy on me. And Jesus stood, and commanded him to be brought unto him: and when he was come near, he asked him, Saying, What wilt thou that I shall do unto thee? And he said, Lord, that I may receive my sight. And Jesus said unto him, Receive thy sight: thy faith hath saved thee. And immediately he received his sight, and followed him, glorifying God: and all the people, when they saw it, gave praise unto God.

Luke 18:35–43

43. Jesus answered and said, Suffer ye thus far. And he touched his ear, and healed him.

Luke 22:51

44. So Jesus came again into Cana of Galilee, where he made the water wine. And there was a certain nobleman, whose son was sick at Capernaum. When he heard that Jesus was come out of Judaea into Galilee, he went unto him, and besought him that he would come down, and heal his son: for he was at the point of death. Then said Jesus unto him, Except ye see signs and wonders, ye will not believe. The nobleman saith unto him, Sir, come down ere my child die. Jesus saith

*unto him, Go thy way; thy son liveth. And the man believed
the word that Jesus had spoken unto him, and he went his
way. And as he was now going down, his servants met him,
and told him, saying, Thy son liveth. Then enquired he of
them the hour when he began to amend. And they said unto
him, Yesterday at the seventh hour the fever left him. So the
father knew that it was at the same hour, in the which Jesus
said unto him, Thy son liveth: and himself believed, and his
whole house. This is again the second miracle that Jesus did,
when he was come out of Judaea into Galilee.*

John 4:46–54

*45. Now there is at Jerusalem by the sheep market a pool,
which is called in the Hebrew tongue Bethesda, having five
porches. In these lay a great multitude of impotent folk, of
blind, halt, withered, waiting for the moving of the water.
For an angel went down at a certain season into the pool, and
troubled the water: whosoever then first after the troubling of
the water stepped in was made whole of whatsoever disease
he had. And a certain man was there, which had an infirmity
thirty and eight years. When Jesus saw him lie, and knew
that he had been now a long time in that case, he saith unto
him, Wilt thou be made whole? The impotent man answered
him, Sir, I have no man, when the water is troubled, to put
me into the pool: but while I am coming, another steppeth
down before me. Jesus saith unto him, Rise, take up thy bed,
and walk. And immediately the man was made whole, and
took up his bed, and walked: and on the same day was the*

sabbath. The Jews therefore said unto him that was cured, It is the sabbath day: it is not lawful for thee to carry thy bed. He answered them, He that made me whole, the same said unto me, Take up thy bed, and walk. Then asked they him, What man is that which said unto thee, Take up thy bed, and walk? And he that was healed wist not who it was: for Jesus had conveyed himself away, a multitude being in that place. Afterward Jesus findeth him in the temple, and said unto him, Behold, thou art made whole: sin no more, lest a worse thing come unto thee. The man departed, and told the Jews that it was Jesus, which had made him whole.

John 5:2–15

46. When he had thus spoken, he spat on the ground, and made clay of the spittle, and he anointed the eyes of the blind man with the clay, And said unto him, Go, wash in the pool of Siloam, (which is by interpretation, Sent) He went his way therefore, and washed, and came seeing.

John 9:6–7

47. When he thus had spoken, he cried with a loud voice, Lazarus, come forth. And he that was dead came forth, bound hand and foot with graveclothes: and his face was bound about with a napkin. Jesus saith unto them, Loose him, and let him go.

John 11:43–44

Receive Jesus as
Your Savior

Choosing to receive Jesus Christ as your Lord and Savior is the most important decision you'll ever make!

God's Word promises, *"That if thou shalt confess with thy mouth the Lord Jesus, and shalt believe in thine heart that God hath raised him from the dead, thou shalt be saved. For with the heart man believeth unto righteousness; and with the mouth confession is made unto salvation"* (Romans 10:9-10). *"For whosoever shall call upon the name of the Lord shall be saved"* (Romans 10:13).

By His grace, God has already done everything to provide salvation. Your part is simply to believe and receive.

Pray out loud, *"Jesus, I confess that You are my Lord and Savior. I believe in my heart that God raised You from the dead. By faith in Your Word, I receive salvation now. Thank You for saving me!"*

The very moment you commit your life to Jesus Christ, the truth of His Word instantly comes to pass in your spirit. Now that you're born again, there's a brand-new you!

Please contact me and let me know that you've prayed to receive Jesus as your Savior or to be filled with the Holy Spirit. I would like to rejoice with you and help you understand more fully what has taken place in your life. I'll send you a free gift that will help you understand and grow in your new relationship with the Lord. *Welcome to your new life!*

Receive the Holy Spirit

As His child, your loving heavenly Father wants to give you the supernatural power you need to live this new life.

"For every one that asketh receiveth; and he that seeketh findeth; and to him that knocketh it shall be opened...how much more shall your heavenly Father give the Holy Spirit to them that ask him?"

Luke 11:10-13

All you have to do is ask, believe, and receive!

Pray, *"Father, I recognize my need for Your power to live this new life. Please fill me with Your Holy Spirit. By faith, I receive it right now! Thank You for baptizing me. Holy Spirit, You are welcome in my life!"*

Congratulations—now you're filled with God's supernatural power!

Some syllables from a language you don't recognize will rise up from your heart to your mouth. (1 Corinthians 14:14.) As you speak them out loud by faith, you're releasing God's power from within and building yourself up in your spirit. (1 Corinthians 14:4.) You can do this whenever and wherever you like.

It doesn't really matter whether you felt anything or not when you prayed to receive the Lord and His Spirit. If you believed in your heart that you received, then God's Word promises that you did. *"Therefore I say unto you, What things soever ye desire, when ye pray, believe that ye receive them, and ye shall have them"* (**Mark 11:24**). God always honors His Word—believe it!

Please contact me and let me know that you've prayed to receive Jesus as your Savior or to be filled with the Holy Spirit. I would like to rejoice with you and help you understand more fully what has taken place in your life. I'll send you a free gift that will help you understand and grow in your new relationship with the Lord. *Welcome to your new life!*

Recommended Teachings

Mentioned in book:

You've Already Got It!

"The Sovereignty of God"

"The Faith of God"

Spirit, Soul & Body

How to Receive a Miracle

A Sure Foundation

Effortless Change

The Believer's Authority

Spiritual Authority

The True Nature of God

God's Kind of Love: The Cure for What Ails Ya

God's Love to You

The War Is Over

Life for Today Study Bible and Commentary—Acts Edition

Others:

God Wants You Well (audio)

Healing Scriptures

Healing Journeys (video)

Hardness of Heart

A Better Way to Pray

What to Do When Your Prayers Seem Unanswered

Niki Ochenski: The Story of a Miracle! (video)

Niki's Healing Testimony

Jodie Stehouwer's Testimony

Stillborn—Krow Family Miracle (video)

Christian Survival Kit

The Book of Job

All Things Work Together for Good

Discover The Keys to Staying Full of God

Endnotes

Introduction

[1]Since this Introduction was first written, I've fought a sinus infection that lasted about three days. This too was stupidity-induced. I had ministered forty-one times one week and then forty times the next. Physically, this wore me out. I was so weak I opened a door to sickness. Faith doesn't always overcome stupidity. I've taken steps to correct this.

Chapter 3

[1]Thayer and Smith, The KJV New Testament Greek Lexicon, "Greek Lexicon entry for Sozo," available from http://www.biblestudytools.com/lexicons/greek/kjv/sozo.html, Strong's #4982.

Chapter 4

[1]Based on information from Thayer and Smith, "Greek Lexicon entry for Anthistemi," Strong's # 436, S.V. "resist," James 4:7.

Chapter 5

[1]Based on definitions from Thayer and Smith, "Greek Lexicon entry for Charakter," available from http://www.studylight.org/lex/grk/view.cgi?number=5481, S.V "image," Hebrews 1:3.

Chapter 7

[1]Thayer and Smith, "Greek Lexicon entry for Aggelos," available from http://www.biblestudytools.com/lexicons/greek/kjv/aggelos.html, S.V. "messenger," 2 Corinthians 12:7.

Chapter 8

[1]See Note 3 at Acts 14:20 and Note 5 at Acts 14:6 of Life for Today Study Bible and Commentary—Acts Edition.

[2]Based on information from Thayer and Smith, "Greek Lexicon entry for Pelikos," available from http/:biblestudytools.com/lexicons/greek/kjv/pelikos.html, S.V. "large," Galatians 6:11.

Chapter 9

[1]Paul's name was "Saul" before the Lord changed it to "Paul." See Acts 9; 13:9.

Chapter 13

[1]A world-renown twentieth century pastor, evangelist, and author who is considered to be the "father" of Christian television. His international ministry is still impacting people today.

About the Author

Andrew's life was forever changed the moment he encountered the supernatural love of God on March 23, 1968. The author of more than thirty books, Andrew has made it his mission for more than five decades to change the way the world sees God.

Andrew's vision is to go as far and deep with the Gospel as possible. His message goes far through the Gospel Truth television and radio program, which is available to nearly half the world's population. The message goes deep through discipleship at Charis Bible College, founded in 1994, which currently has more than seventy campuses and over 6,000 students around the globe. These students will carry on the same mission of changing the way the world sees God. This is Andrew's legacy.

To contact Andrew Wommack please write, e-mail, or call:

Andrew Wommack Ministries, Inc.
P.O. Box 3333 • Colorado Springs, CO 80934-3333
E-mail: info@awmi.net
Helpline Phone (orders and prayer): 719-635-1111
Hours: 4:00 AM to 9:30 PM MST

Andrew Wommack Ministries of Europe
P.O. Box 4392 • WS1 9AR Walsall • England
E-mail: enquiries@awme.net
U.K. Helpline Phone (orders and prayer):
011-44-192-247-3300
Hours: 5:30 AM to 4:00 PM GMT

Or visit him on the Web at: **www.awmi.net**

The Harrison House Vision

Proclaiming the truth and the power
of the Gospel of Jesus Christ with excellence.
Challenging Christians
to live victoriously,
grow spiritually,
know God intimately.